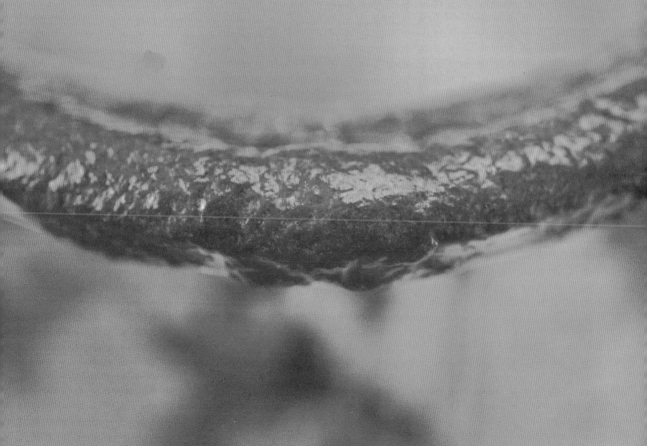

more super juice

michael van straten

more super juice

juicing for health and healing

whitecap

More Super Juice
Michael van Straten

Published in Canada and the United States in 2007 by
Whitecap Books Ltd.
For more information, please contact Whitecap Books Ltd.,
351 Lynn Avenue, North Vancouver,
British Columbia, Canada V7J 2C4.
Visit our website at www.whitecap.ca.

First published in Great Britain in 2007 by Mitchell Beazley,
an imprint of Octopus Publishing Group Limited,
2–4 Heron Quays, London E14 4JP.
© Octopus Publishing Group Limited 2007
Text © Michael van Straten 2007

A CIP catalogue record for this book is available from the
British Library.

ISBN: 978-1-55285-873-8
ISBN: 1-55285-873-1

While all reasonable care has been taken during the preparation
of this edition, neither the publisher, editors nor the author can
accept responsibility for any consequences arising from the use
thereof or from the information contained therein.

More Super Juice is meant to be used as a general recipe book.
While the author believes the recipes it contains are beneficial
to health, the book is in no way intended to replace medical
advice. You are urged to consult a physician about specific
medical complaints and the use of healing herbs and foods
in the treatment thereof.

Commissioning Editor: Rebecca Spry
Executive Art Editor: Nicky Collings
Designer: Geoff Borin
Senior Editor: Hannah McEwen
Copy Editor: Jamie Ambrose
Proofreader: Alyson Silverwood
Photography: Francesca Yorke
Food stylist: Katherine Ibbs
Production: Angela Young
Index: John Noble

Printed and bound by Toppan Printing Company in China
Typeset in FF Kievit

contents

introduction

I have been using juice therapy in my practice for more than 40 years and learned about it from other naturopaths who used it for at least 40 years before I started. Like many of my books, my first juice book, *SuperJuice,* was originally conceived to help my own patients. But when it was first published way back in 1999 I had no idea that it would become a worldwide bestseller. Most of the existing books on juicing were worthy but equally dull; it was *SuperJuice* that broke the mold and made juicing fun and exciting as well as healthy. I'm sure that *SuperJuice* was a major factor in the huge expansion of interest in juice therapy, the dramatic increase in sales of juicers' and the mushrooming of juice bars in city centers everywhere.

Now that so many of you have got the juice habit and have discovered for yourselves both the pleasures and the benefits of juicing, I think it's time to be a little more adventurous. Here in *More Super Juice* you'll find some fairly conventional recipes as well as some that I've devised for very specific purposes that may sound a trifle odd. Don't knock them until you've tried them, because even the strangest juices taste a lot better than they sound.

On one of my radio programs recently, the station sent a radio car and a reporter to the home of a lady who'd called a few weeks earlier complaining of chronic fatigue after a bout of severe food poisoning. I persuaded her to get her juicer out of the cabinet, where it had sat for two years, and sent her some recipes. Within two weeks, she'd called the station and said she felt fantastic and was never going to put her juicer back in the cabinet again. When our surprise reporter turned up on her doorstep with a bag of mixed fruits and veggies, I talked her through a couple of unusual combinations and the whole family joined in the tasting. Even her teenage son (who hates *all* vegetables) asked for a second glass of the beet recipe!

The great thing about owning a juicer is that you can put almost anything that grows through the machine. It's the perfect way to get extra nutrients out of the bits you might otherwise throw away: the outside leaves of the cabbage or lettuce, the red pepper in the bottom of your vegetable rack, the Brussels sprouts the kids won't eat, the half an onion left over from a recipe—it's all food for free. There are no rules, no conventions; just let your imagination run riot. Of course you'll make some mistakes and the results will taste disgusting, but when you come up with a really fabulous combination, write it down in your own book.

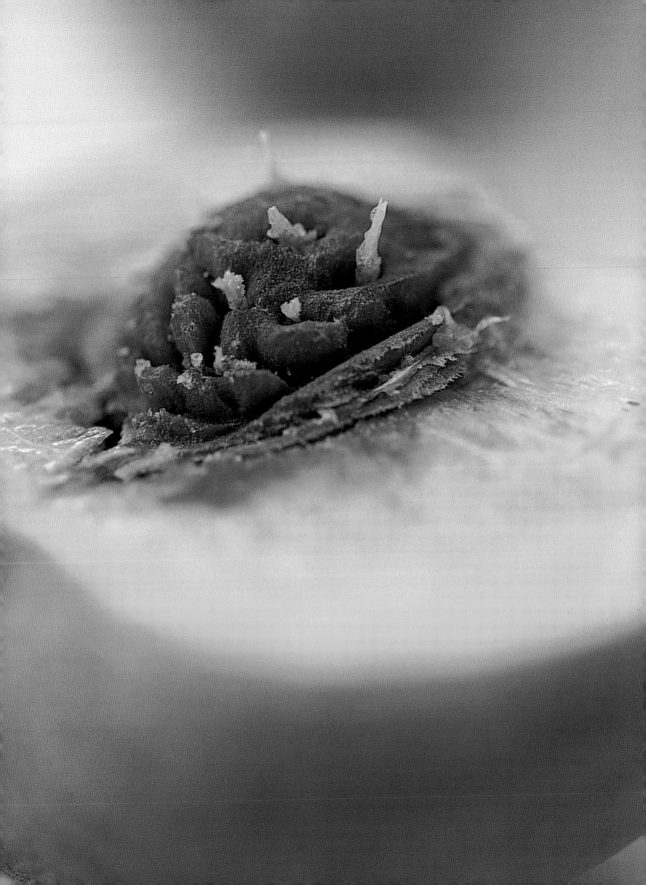

how to use this book

First and foremost, *More Super Juice* is a recipe book: a collection of different ways of combining ingredients. Some recipes are conventional, some are unusual, and others are rather strange, but they're all here for a purpose—don't dismiss them just because they seem "alien" at first sight! You won't find meaningless figures in *More Super Juice*. Instead, simple descriptions show the vitamins and minerals in one 1 cup of juice. All recipes make at least one glass, and some make more than one.

Other than where specifically stated, all relative proportions listed in recipes are approximate. In addition, quantities of ingredients will vary according to size, variety and ripeness; some apples are bigger than others, after all! With a bit of practice, you'll soon become expert at judging how many carrots or apples yield 1 cup of juice.

The book is divided into two sections. The first (and largest) is devoted to enhancing the life you already lead. It begins with recipes for power and vitality juices, followed by a cleansing section that shows how to detox your system quickly and successfully. There are also juices designed specifically to improve your mood and memory, enhance and protect your immune system—even boost your sex drive. Booze juices, slimming juices and shakes and smoothies follow.

The second part of the book, Super Detox on page 124, deals with the curative powers of juicing. It shows you how to rid your body of all the harmful elements derived from modern living, and includes detox diets for energy, radiance, brain-boosting, cleansing, immunity, and healing. The second section concludes with the "drink yourself better" tables on page 138, allowing you to choose a juice to treat specific illnesses. Finally, on page 142, you'll find an ORAC table that will help you identify the foods that are best for helping your body neutralize free radicals. Simply by minimizing the level of free radicals (the chemicals at the core of the aging process), you help protect your body against heart disease, strokes, many forms of cancer and degenerative diseases such as arthritis, maintain good vision, and help every organ and system in your body to work at maximum efficiency.

how to juice

The whole point of juicing is to get the maximum amount of vitamins, minerals, enzymes, and phytochemicals out of food and into your body. For this reason, buy organic produce whenever possible—especially if you're juicing for babies and small children—and make sure your produce is in peak condition.

Wash all produce thoroughly, scrubbing tough-skinned varieties with a soft brush. All fruits and vegetables should be juiced with their skins, except where otherwise stated. Non-organic produce should be washed in a solution of one teaspoon of dish washing liquid to four cups of warm water and then rinsed thoroughly; this removes most external chemical residues. Don't prepare and chop up produce before you need it as this causes vitamin loss. When juicing small quantities of ingredients—six mint leaves, a small piece of gingerroot, a few sage leaves—wrap them in one of the other ingredients first. When using ice, put it in the blender with a little water and switch on for a few seconds before adding the other ingredients.

juicing kit
There are many types of juicers (and I've tried most of them) at prices ranging from $40 to $1000+. If you've never juiced before, start with an inexpensive machine. You have two basic choices.

The generally less expensive type is a centrifugal juicer, that whizzes the fruits or veggies round on a serrated blade, allowing the juice to strain through a filter. The pulp is either retained inside the machine or thrown out into a separate container. For two or three glasses it doesn't make much difference, but for larger amounts you'll have to stop and remove the pulp to clear the filter before you start again. The juicer I use every day is the SuperJuicer—in which I have absolutely no commercial interest. It's a centrifugal machine that throws out the pulp, has a high extraction rate and is easy to clean.

The second type is a masticating juicer, that crushes the produce between special rollers. These work at lower speeds and much more juice is extracted, leaving a very dry pulp that is automatically extruded by the machine. These tend to be the larger, heavier and most expensive pieces of equipment, but they're no doubt the Rolls-Royce of juicers if you're really serious. In my opinion, the best models are The Champion and The Green Machine.

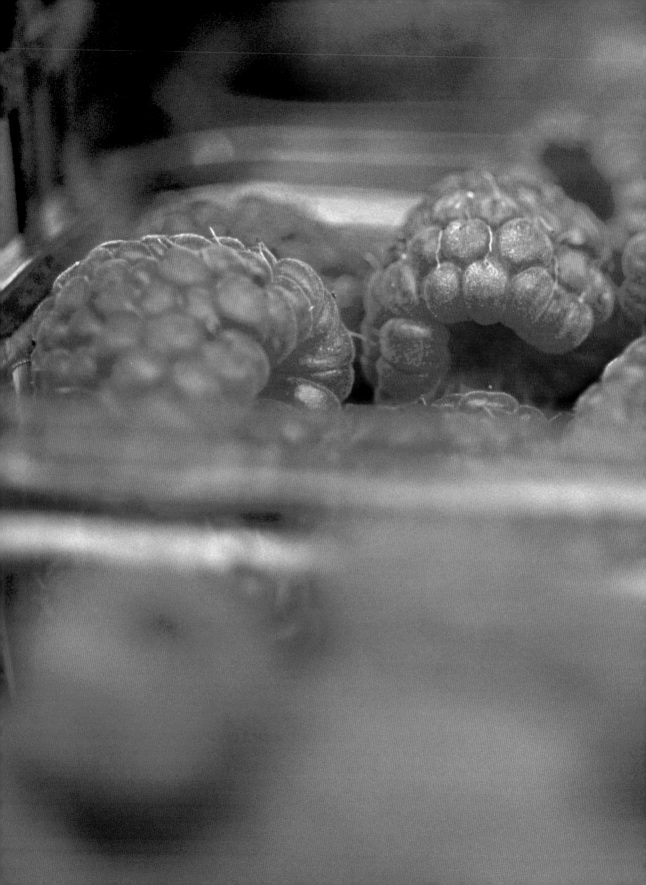

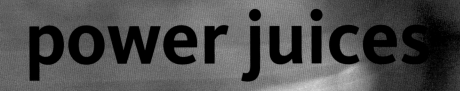

power juices

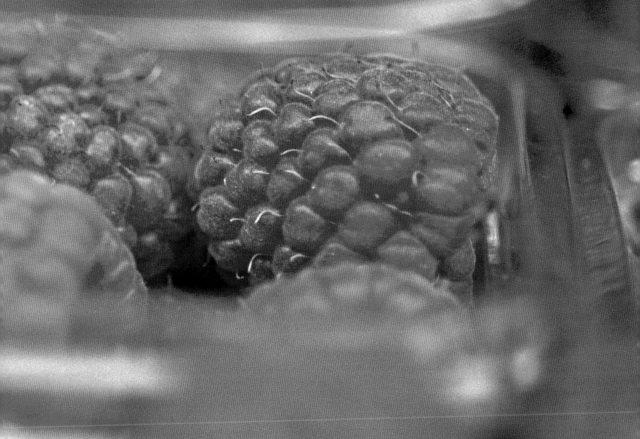

One of the most important chemical processes to take place in the body is the conversion of food into energy that can then be used to power physical and mental activity. In fact, this process is the body's generating plant; without sufficient foods that increase the availability of power, the body winds down and loses energy, leaving you tired, sluggish, and not at your best intellectual level.

Eating well is, of course, a basic necessity, but unfortunately the ever-increasing consumption of refined carbohydrates and high-fat, high-sugar convenience foods can create a constant drain on your power output. One part of the problem is the amount of high glycemic index (GI) foods in the modern diet. White bread, cakes, cookies, white rice, huge amounts of sugar (up to 11 teaspoons in a can of soda) and all the other refined carbohydrates that abound in processed foods are the root of the problem. They're very quickly broken down in the body, releasing sugar into the bloodstream—that results in the pancreas producing excessive quantities of insulin. The insulin breaks down the sugar, but once that's all gone it sets to work on the body's stores of energy.

The end result is this constant swinging from high levels of blood sugar to very low, and it's this hypoglycemia (low blood sugar) that stimulates a desperate craving for more sugar. The grand finale is an ever-increasing dependency on a high-sugar, high-refined carbohydrate fix, but this only serves to perpetuate the problem. Once established, this pattern is the trigger for "Syndrome X," or insulin dependency, that leads to non-insulin-dependent diabetes (NIDD). Historically, NIDD has always been known as late-onset diabetes to differentiate it from the type of diabetes that is present at birth or that develops very early on in life in those affected. Tragically, we're now seeing increasing numbers of eight-, nine- and ten-year-olds with NIDD.

The way to generate power and avoid NIDD is to make sure that most of the carbohydrates you consume are the complex carbohydrates, that have a low GI. These come from wholegrain cereals, oats, rye, barley, beans, peas, lentils, nuts, and seeds. They release their energy slowly, so they don't trigger a huge release of insulin. They're also mostly excellent sources of both soluble and insoluble fiber that are vital for good digestion and the reduction of cholesterol levels.

In addition to a healthy diet, the juices in this chapter will all help improve your power and energy, both mental and physical. What's more, they taste terrific!

pears 2
soy milk 3/4 cup
banana 1, peeled
plain yogurt 1/2 cup
ground cinnamon 1 generous pinch
ice cubes 1 handful

sweet pear

This kaleidoscope of nutrients will not only help generate energy but is also good for the muscles, bones, and hormones. Probiotics in the yogurt improve digestion and boost resistance, and the latest research on cinnamon shows that it helps to regulate insulin levels in diabetics.

vital statistics

Bananas are a rich source of potassium, that is essential for muscle effort. The yogurt provides calcium for strong bones, while soy milk is rich in phytoestrogens to aid the absorption of calcium, and the sweet pears provide energy-releasing fruit sugar.

cucumber 1 large

celery 1 stick, with leaves

lemon 1, with peel if thin-skinned

lime 1, peeled unless key lime

green energy

This really is a green juice, but if you think mixing cucumber with citrus fruit juice is strange, you'll be pleasantly surprised by the taste. It's not hugely rich in nutrients but is very cleansing and has no adverse effects on blood-sugar levels.

vital statistics

Lots of **vitamin C** and protective **bioflavonoids** from the citrus fruits are combined with muscle-boosting **potassium** in the celery. This is a mildly diuretic juice that helps elimination and the relief of joint pain, making movement more comfortable.

potatoes 2 medium
apples 2, sweet (such as Pink Lady)
mint 1 good sprig

apple of your eye

This juice provides a fantastic combination of energy-giving starch from the potatoes and fruit sugar from the apples. You may think it sounds disgusting, but don't knock it until you've tried it.

vital statistics

Both potato starch and fruit sugar are broken down by the body to release energy, and although they don't have a GI as low as the complex carbs in legumes, it's a lot lower than spoons of sugar in your tea. The **essential oils** from the mint leaves helps improve digestion of the nutrients.

leek 1 small
cucumber ½
garlic 2 cloves
cilantro 1 handful of leaves
beet 1 large

welsh wizard

Leeks have a long history stretching back into ancient Rome, where they were eaten by the emperors for their health-giving properties. Together with the garlic (a member of the same family: the all-powerful alliums) and the beet, they make an attractive and very savory juice with a high energy potential.

vital statistics

Although not that rich in general nutrients, leeks contain **plant chemicals** that encourage the elimination of uric acid and so reduce the discomfort of arthritic joints. The beet is a blood tonic and an excellent source of slow-release energy, so this juice is both pain-relieving and energizing.

pineapple 1 small, peeled and sliced
kiwi fruit 2
celery 1 stick, with leaves
cucumber ½
cilantro 1 handful

pineapple power

Once a pineapple is harvested it's as ripe as it's ever going to be. After that, it just rots, so the old wives' tale of pulling out the leaves to see if it's ripe is simply not true. The only test is its weight: if it feels heavy for its size, then it has a high sugar content and will be ripe, sweet, and juicy.

vital statistics

Both the pineapple and kiwi fruit provide slow-release energy in the form of fruit sugars. The celery is a good source of potassium, that is important for muscle strength. Don't peel the cucumber before juicing as you lose its protective betacarotene.

sweet potatoes 2 medium

celery 3 sticks

watermelon ¼, peeled and seeded

carrots 4 large, topped and tailed, peeled if not organic

peanuts ¼ cup, chopped and toasted

southern super-fit

Sweet potato, peanuts, and watermelon are traditional foods from the American Deep South. Combined in this drink, they provide both the instant and slower-release energy that athletes require. It doesn't matter whether you are aiming for the Olympics or just thinking of next Saturday's kick-about in the local park; both will need instant and sustained effort. So juice the fruit and veggies first, then sprinkle with the peanuts.

vital statistics

Peanuts supply **protein** and **oils**, both of which are digested slowly so they provide a sustained release of energy. The melon and carrots contain **sugars** that are able to give you an instant burst of energy for the explosive activity needed in most sport. The **vitamin C** and **carotenes** help the repair and restoration needed after any intensive physical activity.

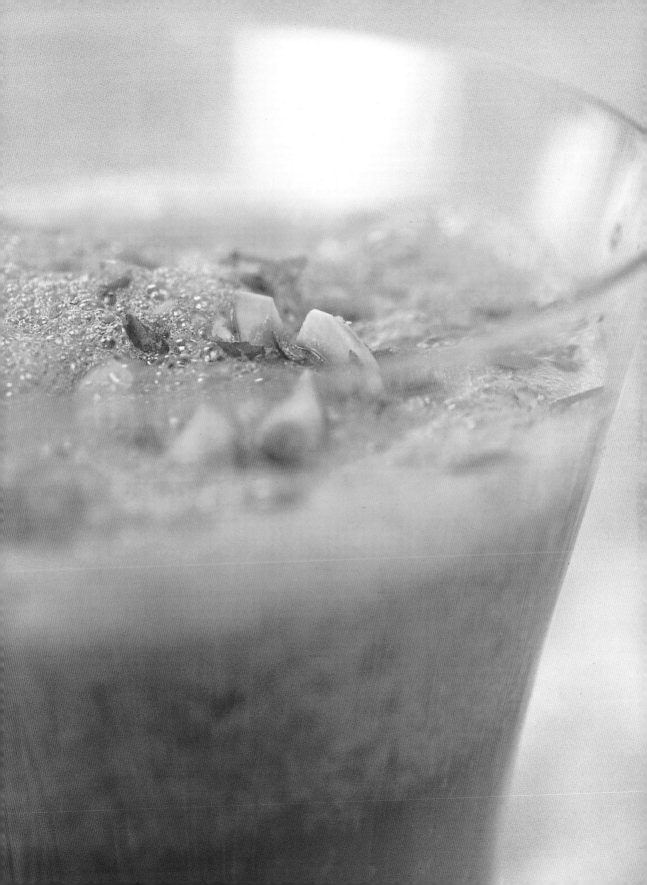

cherries 1/2 cup, pitted
pears 3
apple 1
celery 2 sticks, with leaves
kiwi fruit 2
celery seeds 1/2 teaspoon, crushed

joint pack

Here's a recipe that helps maintain mobility by taking care of your joints. Historically, both cherries and celery have been used in folk medicine for the relief of joint pain. In this recipe they're made delicious by the addition of the other fruit.

vital statistics

As long ago as ancient Greece, traditional physicians valued cherries as a treatment for arthritis and gout. They're rich in bioflavonoids, potassium, and vitamin C with virtually no sodium. Celery, although poor in general nutrients, is an excellent diuretic that helps reduce the levels of inflammatory uric acid in the joints. The seeds are a traditional treatment for arthritis and gout, and provide flavor as well as medicinal benefits.

carrots 4, topped and tailed, peeled if not organic
strawberries 8, hulled
tomatoes 2
watercress 1 bunch
parsley 1 small handful, with leaves and stalks
kale 4 leaves, including stems

cress to impress

Power needs movement. If your mobility is restricted by painful joints, this strange-sounding mixture of fruits and vegetables really will help to ease the pain, improve mobility, and allow you to utilize your body's innate energy.

vital statistics

As well as the normal nutritional content you'd expect (like betacarotene and vitamin C), the strawberries help reduce joint inflammation. The phytochemicals in kale are both protective and anti-inflammatory, and the parsley is a gentle diuretic that helps increase the excretion of joint-damaging uric acid.

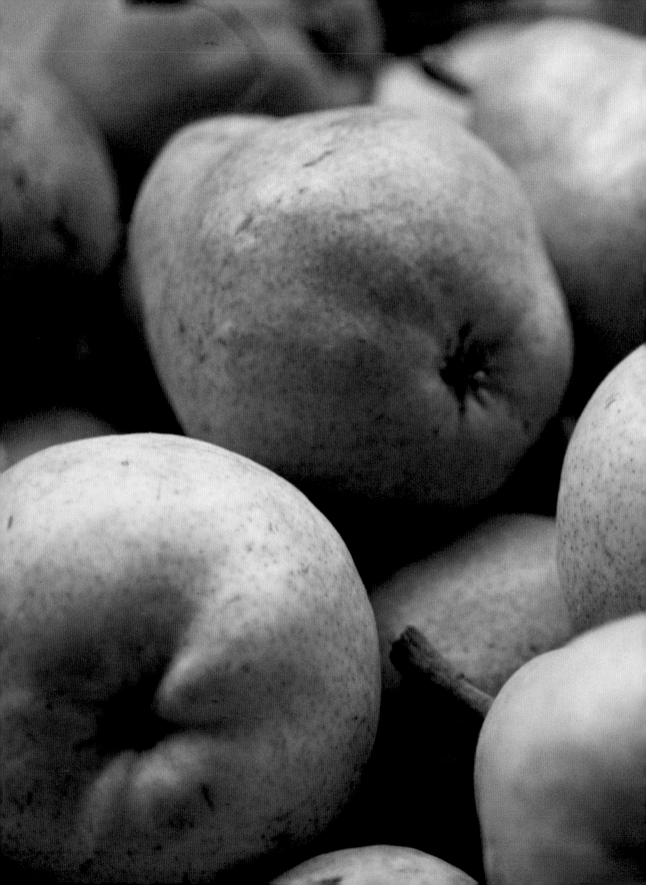

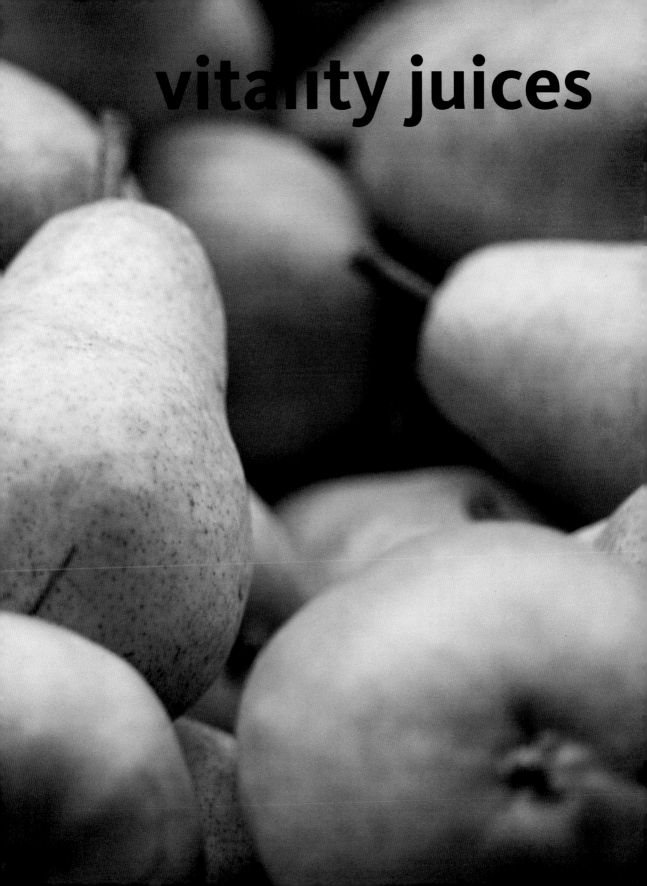

vitality juices

Millions of people all over the world wake up every morning unable to comprehend how they're going to struggle through the rest of the day. Fatigue, tiredness, and lack of vitality make up the most commonly reported symptoms in the UK population. Almost 40 percent listed fatigue in a survey of health problems they'd recently suffered. Although 90 percent of the people surveyed felt they were frequently lacking in vitality, 70 percent of them did nothing about it. They didn't change their diets, they didn't take a tonic, they didn't even see their family doctor.

Anyone living with a constant lack of vitality and chronic fatigue should undergo a medical consultation just to rule out the possibility of underlying illness. Once you've been told that there's no apparent reason for your problem, you can take matters into your own hands, improve your diet, and use these eight vitality juices on a regular basis.

It's natural that everyone loses their spark at some time or another. Late nights, a hard day at work, family problems, travel frazzle, or simply needing a break away from it all... they can all grind away at your vitality and leave you a victim of chronic fatigue. It's true that total lack of vitality and constant tiredness are common symptoms of depression, anxiety, and other psychological problems, but let's face it: if you are constantly exhausted, you're going to get depressed—you can get caught in a downward spiral where the cause becomes physical, as well as mental.

Anemia, thyroid problems, chronic pain, viral infections, a poorly designed vegetarian or vegan diet, or just plain bad eating can all lie at the root of the problem. Unfortunately, this can turn into a vicious circle of bad eating, which leaves you lacking in vitality so that you don't have the energy to go shopping; you then eat more junk food, more takeouts and become even more poorly nourished, draining away whatever vitality you've got left. What you need is a simple, well-balanced and widely varied diet that doesn't avoid any whole food groups—one that doesn't allow for faddy ideas or the latest crank peddling bogus nutrition and advising the whole world to live on wheatgrass juice, energy powders, pills, and colonic irrigation.

So ignore the charlatans and the cranks and eat good, wholesome, and delicious food. Start with these fabulous juices.

mango 1, peeled, pit removed

pawpaw 1, seeded, flesh scooped out

pineapple 2 thick slices, peeled

passion fruit 2, flesh scooped out

lime 1, peeled unless key lime

tropical treasure

Vitality just pours out of this treasure chest of tropical fruits. They look good, they smell great and they taste fantastic—and you'll start to feel better after the first glass. The great thing about pineapple and pawpaw is that they both contain healing enzymes that you can get only from the fresh fruit or freshly made juices.

vital statistics

Contains lots of good fruit sugars for instant energy from all the fruits. Enzymes from the mango, pawpaw, and pineapple improve digestion and help you extract optimum nutrition from the food you eat. This juice also provides two days' worth of betacarotene and around four days' worth of vitamin C in every single glass.

pink grapefruit* 1, peeled, but with pith
grapefruit* 1, ordinary, peeled, but with pith
oranges 2, Seville or blood, peeled, but with pith
clementines 2, peeled
lime 1, peeled unless key lime

citrus symphony

A great, clean-tasting mixture of these citrus fruits with a hint of bitterness from the oranges and tartness from the limes make this a brilliant apéritif. Your gastric juices will be working overtime before you're halfway through the glass.

*If taking prescribed medicines, consult your doctor before drinking large amounts of grapefruit juice.

vital statistics

You'll get nearly a week's worth of **vitamin C**—but just as importantly, lots of protective **bioflavonoids** plus the bitter **phytochemicals** in the orange and grapefruit pith, that stimulate the flow of digestive juices and improve the digestion of any food that follows.

black grapes 2½ cups
comice pear 1 large
guava 1, peeled
honey 2 teaspoons
whole milk 1¼ cups
apricots 4 dried
almonds 2 teaspoons, ground

instant energy

There are times when your vitality needs a short sharp kick up the backside—and here's the juice to do it. This complex mixture of fruits, milk, honey, and nuts will start restoring your vitality with an instant energy boost within 10 minutes of drinking it, and it will last for two or three hours. Simply juice the fruit and whiz it with everything else in a blender.

vital statistics

Instant energy comes from the honey, slightly slower-release energy from the grapes, pear, and guava, then from the apricots, and slow-release energy from the proteins in the milk and almonds. This smoothie is also extremely rich in a whole range of essential nutrients and won't trigger short-term sugar cravings that get you on the see-saw of rapidly rising and falling blood-sugar levels.

pomegranate 1, seeds and flesh only
pears 3
dessert apples 2
blueberries ⅔ cup

seeds of life

Quintessential vitality from the hundreds of seeds in the pomegranate makes this a valuable juice. From all the recent fuss about this fruit, you may think that it is an amazing new product from a GM lab, but this couldn't be further from the truth. The pomegranate has an ancient history. Used as a medicine for thousands of years, it is also thought to be a powerful aphrodisiac in many cultures.

vital statistics

Enjoy the energy from the natural sugars as well as the enormous protective antioxidant chemicals from the natural coloring in the pomegranate and the blueberries. There is also a good supply of vitamin C and carotenoids.

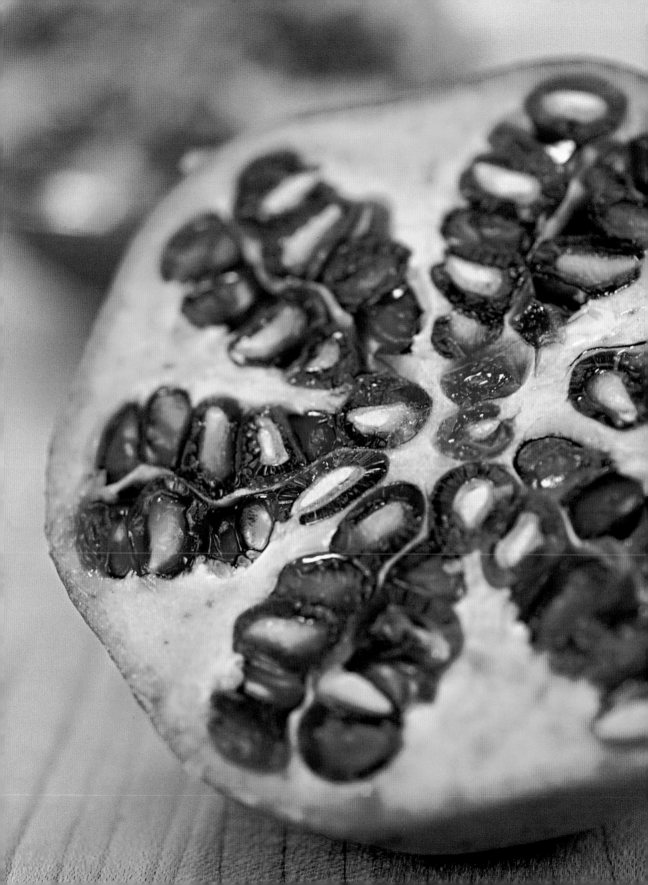

pears 3 such as Beurre Hardy
white grapes 2¹/₂ cups, seedless

the perfect pear

You'd automatically think of apples and pears, but grapes and pears are also a natural combination—just juice them all together and enjoy. Don't add ice or chill as you'll lose the wonderful aroma. Any of the really sweet, juicy pears will do, but if you can get some of the Beurre Hardy variety, you'll be amazed at their flavor. Why not plant your own? This variety has been around since 1820, and is an early ripener in mid-September and, as its name suggests, it's hardy and grows almost anywhere.

vital statistics

Lots of **natural sugars** from the pears and grapes make this a real instant vitality pair. Pears are also a rich source of **pectin**, the natural fiber that helps lower cholesterol and improve digestion.

cox's apples 3
russet apples 2
cooking apple 1
raspberries 1½ cups

special apple energizer

In recent years, single-variety and named apple mixtures have been commercially available as bottled juices. Save yourself a fortune, avoid any additives and get maximum nutrition by juicing your own. Use any combination of apple varieties you like, but the ones named here are only available in the early fall, when they are at their prime. It's this time of the year when the second crop of late raspberries also appears in the markets, and they're full of flavor and natural sugars.

vital statistics

Mixing the dessert and cooking apples provides a good content of fruit sugars and the soluble fiber pectin, that together give a nice, gentle energy release. Adding the raspberries, which have a high sugar content if they're ripe, will give you a quick burst of vitality before the other components kick in.

strawberries 3 cups, hulled

blueberries 1¹/₃ cups

figs 2

pear 1

lemon ¹/₂, unpeeled if thin-skinned

blue strawberries

Figs come very high up the list of vitality foods. As Adam and Eve used fig leaves to cover their modesty, they must have eaten the figs—and I've never understood why they bothered with the apple! For many, the fig is a sacred tree; the very earliest of Olympians were fed masses of fresh figs for vitality, strength, and stamina. Juiced together with the other fruit, this is a fabulous-tasting drink with a maximum vitality rating.

vital statistics

As well as containing a natural anti-cancer agent, healing enzymes, and a chemical that improves digestion, figs are an excellent source of iron, potassium, betacarotene, and energy. Strawberries and blueberries are also highly protective against many diseases and, thanks to their high fructose content, a valuable source of sustainable energy and vitality.

spinach 1 generous handful of washed leaves

apples 3 sweet such as Fiesta

carrots 3 large, topped and tailed, peeled if not organic

the gardener's tonic

Have you noticed that, although he's over 70, Popeye still doesn't wear glasses? That's all down to the spinach. Though the iron is not easily absorbed, it's a rich source of the eye-protective nutrients that prevent age-related macular degeneration (AMD). You really need to use sweet apples for this juice to offset the slight bitterness of the spinach leaves. Juice the rolled-up spinach leaves first so that the apples and carrots push all of it through the machine to extract maximum benefit.

vital statistics

Here again it's the natural sugars in the apples and carrots that provide the vitality boost, but you also get betacarotene, lutein, and zeaxanthine, all of which are vital for night vision and long-term eye health.

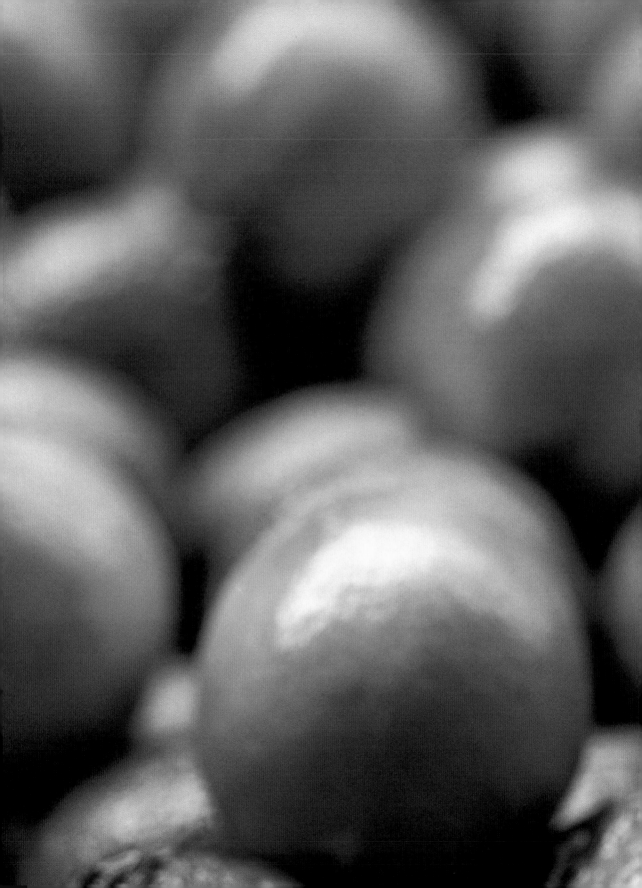

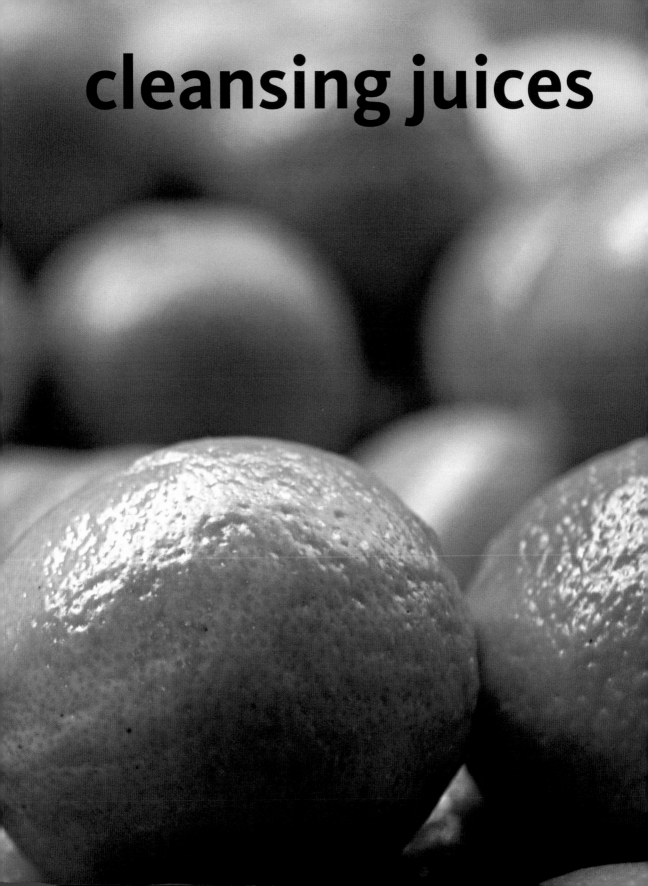

cleansing juices

Fed on a reasonable diet and left to their own devices, the body's cleansing systems work perfectly well for themselves. But how often does this actually happen? There are many things that affect your body's normal function, but amazingly there are really only two factors you can't control. It isn't possible to choose your parents, so the genes you inherit and the influence they have are beyond your control. The other uncontrollable factor is an act of God: you can't foresee them, you can't influence them, and there's no way you can control them. Aside from these exceptions, however, most other health problems encountered during a normal lifetime are more or less in your own hands—and that includes maintaining, assisting, and improving your body's cleansing abilities.

I've been practising as an osteopath, naturopath, acupuncturist, and nutritional consultant for well over 40 years, so there aren't many things people do to damage their health that I haven't seen before. But in spite of all those years and many thousands of patients, I still find it extraordinary that most people think nothing about their nutrition and lifestyle and the serious effect these factors have on both mind and body.

Yet people at the opposite end of the spectrum, although rarer, are still just as worrying. These are the often intelligent, educated, yet gullible people who are completely taken in by every new health fad that they read about in the papers or see some new guru talking about on TV. They are in the minority, but they sometimes worry me more than the people who never give a second thought to their health and wellbeing.

My advice is to beware of extreme diets, the expensive latest "natural" health products that have a secret formula and can only be bought from one particular place. All too often these extreme ideas are focused purely on cleansing the body; I've seen patients who've been hooked on some form of extreme diet, who have excluded whole food groups with no good reason, who believe they're suffering from some new and previously undiscovered health problem, and who seek the answer by using all manner of laxatives, purgatives, and other cleansing supplements that are likely to do much more harm than good.

Extreme measures aren't necessary if, most of the time, you eat sensibly, indulge moderately, and follow a reasonably healthy lifestyle. What you do some of the time doesn't really matter much; however, the cleansing process can benefit from the occasional kick-start, so here are eight interesting juices you can use whenever you feel the need.

raspberries 1¹/₃ cups
blueberries 1¹/₃ cups
black currants ¹/₂ cup
strawberries ²/₃ cup, hulled
lemons 2, unpeeled if thin-skinned

purple lady

This juice is best when strawberries are in season, as that's when they have their highest nutrient content. Pick your own or buy locally grown varieties whenever possible—these delicate fruits don't travel well. Often thought of as too acidic and bad for arthritics, the truth is the exact opposite. In fact, these succulent fruits have an amazing cleansing ability that increases the body's elimination of the uric acid that irritates inflamed joints.

vital statistics

Super-rich in vitamin C, rich in vitamins A and E, and a good source of potassium. Due to the high content of natural salicylates (aspirin-like substances) and ellagic acid in strawberries, this juice is a natural, safe painkiller (especially good for all forms of arthritis) as well as being a powerful anti-cancer mixture. The fruit acids from the berries and currants all help with the cleansing functions, and the high content of pectin in the strawberries also helps eliminate cholesterol and stimulate digestion.

peaches 2, pitted
apricots 4, pitted
yellow plums 4, pitted
pineapple ½, peeled
star fruit 1

tooty fruity

Here's a delicious cleansing juice given a slightly unusual flavor by the addition of star fruit (carambola). Originally a native of Java and Southeast Asia, this attractive fruit is another natural digestive stimulant. Before juicing, carefully slice off and discard the brown edges along the ribs of the star fruit, as this is where oxalic acid, which may interfere with calcium absorption, tends to concentrate.

vital statistics

Contains **cleansing enzymes** from the pineapple and a gentle acidity from the apricots and plums which adds to the overall cleansing properties of this juice. Peaches and apricots contain high levels of **betacarotene,** which are important for healthy skin and natural immunity.

apples 4 crisp (such as Cox's)
cooking apples 2 Lord Derby if possible
fresh mint 20 leaves
cloves ½ teaspoon, ground
turmeric ½ teaspoon, ground

prevention or cure?

There's no doubt that an ounce of prevention is worth a ton of cure, and this recipe is a great example. The combination of spices, mint, and all the apples is not only a huge boost of protective antioxidants but also an effective cleansing booster. Juice the apples and mint, and stir in the cloves and turmeric before drinking.

vital statistics

The mint leaves are one of the best digestive aids and relieve hyperacidity, improve the efficiency of digestion, and help to reduce any undigested residue that's sometimes difficult to excrete. Turmeric is one of the most effective protective spices that helps prevent stomach cancer, and the combination of the fiber, malic and tartaric acids in the apples also stimulates digestion and helps the breakdown and elimination of fats.

mangoes 2, peeled and pitted
hot red chili pepper ½ small, seeded

hot mango

Although you may not think of combining chilies and mangoes, it's actually quite a common combination in Asian cooking. In Ayurvedic medicine, food is seen as an integral part of therapy, and combining hot and sweet is a typical approach in this type of healing.

vital statistics

Juicing the mangoes with the chili pepper provides an extremely rich collection of vital nutrients, particularly vitamins A, C, and E, along with some potassium, iron, and other B vitamins. Here they're used as a vehicle to carry scalding-hot capsaicin from the chili and make it more palatable. It's this ingredient that stimulates the cleansing process and exerts its specific effects on the sinuses and digestive system to boost elimination and cleansing.

apples 4 sweet (such as worcester)

carrots 2 large, topped and tailed, peeled if not organic

white cabbage ¼, cut in wedges

red cabbage ¼, cut in wedges

more than skin deep

Carrots, apples, and cabbage sound like coleslaw, but when all are juiced together, the end result is a sweet, peppery juice with a complex and unusual flavor and a great cleansing effect.

vital statistics

This cleansing juice works in a variety of ways. The apple fiber helps remove cholesterol. The white cabbage juice provides cancer-fighting indoles, and the red cabbage juice is much richer in betacarotenes. The overall effect is to stimulate bowel function and improve elimination.

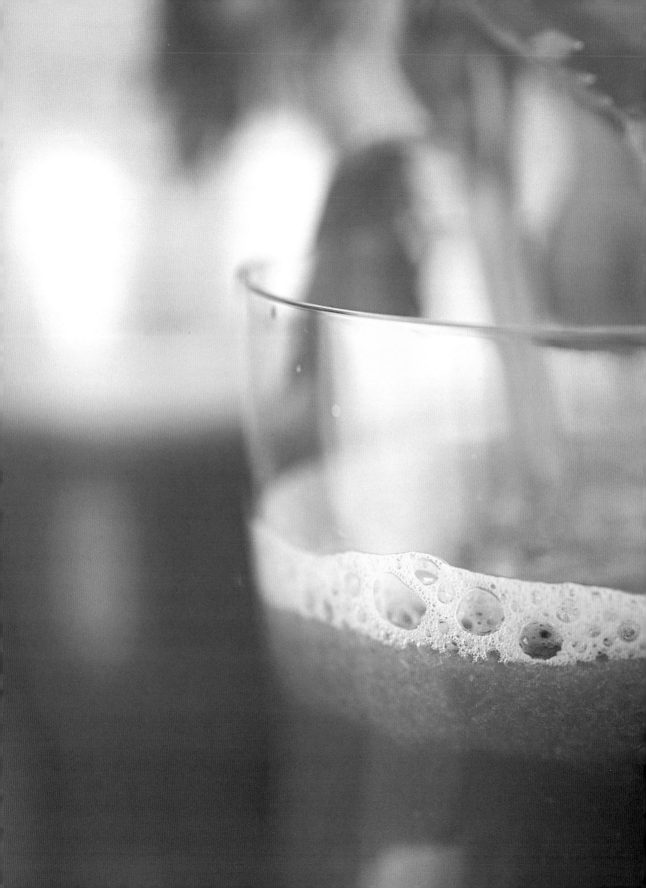

celery 3 sticks, with leaves
fennel ½ bulb
cucumber 1
sage 6 fresh leaves
scallions 2, green part and bulb
worcestershire sauce 1 dash

celery surprise

This cleansing juice works because it combines a number of diuretic, liver-stimulating and antibacterial ingredients. It really helps if you can find a proper old-fashioned bunch of celery with all its leaves on rather than the washed and trimmed supermarket variety. The same is true for the fennel bulb, as the frond-like leaves also help increase fluid elimination. Simply juice all the ingredients and serve with a dash of Worcestershire sauce.

vital statistics

Celery and (to a lesser extent) cucumber are both mild diuretics and help the body eliminate surplus fluid. Fennel and sage both improve fat digestion by stimulating the gall bladder and increasing the flow of bile, that breaks fat down into tiny globules that are more easily digested. Sage and scallions are both effective antibacterial plants that help protect against infection.

celeriac root 7 oz
horseradish root 1 inch
flat-leaf parsley 1 handful
celery 2 sticks, with leaves
cucumber 1/2
watercress 1 generous handful
celery seeds 1/2 teaspoon, crushed

new spring-clean tonic

Celery, parsley, and celeriac are all natural mild diuretics that stimulate a slight increase in urinary output, which helps get rid of excessive fluids without disturbing the balance between sodium and potassium. Just put all the vegetables through the juicer and sprinkle the crushed celery seeds on each glass to serve.

vital statistics

Horseradish is regarded as little more than a condiment to go with your roast beef or smoked fish, but for centuries it has been cultivated as a medicinal herb with a history that predates the Bible. As a **cleanser**, it clears the sinuses and helps get rid of infected phlegm. It also has powerful **antibacterial** properties that contribute to its cleansing power. Mixed with this generally **diuretic** juice and the mustard oils in watercress, it makes a powerful combination.

jerusalem artichokes 4
carrots 4, topped and tailed, peeled if not organic
radishes 4
cilantro 1 handful

fast tox

Here's a pretty instant solution to the previous night's overindulgence. Whether it's too much fatty food, too much cream on the dessert, too many chocolates, or just a good old-fashioned hangover, this combination will rapidly encourage the body to get rid of the waste products that are making you feel so awful.

vital statistics

The soluble fiber inulin in Jerusalem artichokes stimulates bowel function, provides prebiotic food for essential gut bacteria, and helps the body break down and eliminate surplus cholesterol. The radishes are a very specific stimulant of the gall bladder, helping it to pump more bile into the stomach to improve the digestion of an excessive consumption of fat. Juiced together with the cilantro, you have a valuable and effective cleansing juice.

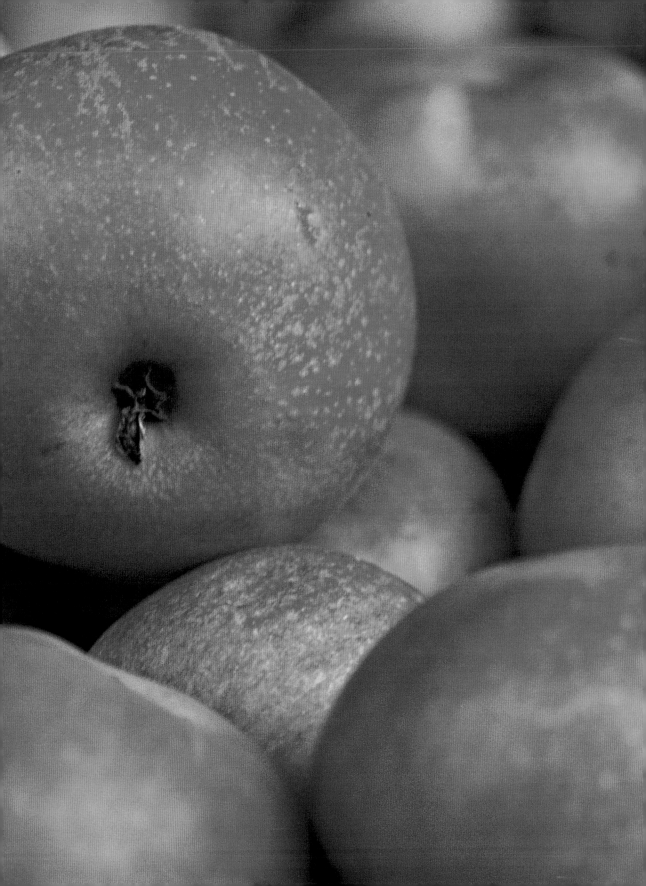

good-mood juices

Since the dawn of time, man has understood the link between food, drink, and mood—and it's not hard to distinguish between good and bad outcomes. Just think back to the dreadful depression you had when you woke with your first hangover. Think how low you feel after a long day at work and a difficult journey home when you haven't stopped for lunch. And what about the anxiety and jitters when you've had your tenth cup of coffee in one morning?

A poor diet can have a disastrous impact on the way we feel, and there are endless research papers that unravel the links between lack of essential nutrients and low mood, depression, and other psychological problems. It's no surprise that, just like all the other parts of the body, the brain and nervous system will only do their jobs when they are adequately supplied with the nutrients they need.

Although the link between deficiencies and mood disruption has been known for years, it has taken generations for the scientific world to accept that better food produces good moods more effectively than taking pills. You may believe that your bad-mood problems are all in the mind, but in many situations there is no need to go through life on tranquilizers or antidepressants.

We know how anemia, which causes so many health problems, can be improved by diet, and how many people—especially young women and teenagers—are desperately short of the key mineral iron. Low mood and depression can be directly linked to low iron intake and even borderline anemia. Women suffering the emotional lows of premenstrual syndrome (PMS) can also boost their mood by eating more foods rich in zinc, magnesium, and vitamin B_6.

These eight juices will all help boost your mood, but you also need to look at your general diet and make sure that it contains plenty of grapes, bananas, and berries; oats, buckwheat, barley, wheat germ, and rye; yeast extracts, molasses, shellfish, sardines, liver, and beef; sunflower and pumpkin seeds, walnuts, almonds, and flaxseeds; asparagus, beet, spinach, endive, and peppers; basil, lemon balm, mint, sage, oregano, nutmeg, cinnamon, and dark chocolate.

blueberries $2/3$ cup
strawberries $1/3$ cup, hulled
cranberries $1/4$ cup
wheatgerm 2 teaspoons
flaxseed oil 1 teaspoon
banana 1
soy milk $1 1/4$ cups

perfect balance

To maintain emotional balance and good mood, enjoy this complex mixture of berries with wheatgerm and soy milk. Together, the ingredients provide a wide spread of good-mood nutrients that will also help build strong bones and boost your natural immunity. Juice all the berries and blend with the other ingredients to serve.

vital statistics

A juice with enormous quantities of protective plant chemicals, B vitamins from the wheatgerm, potassium and B_6 from banana, brain-essential fatty acids from the flaxseed oil, and phytoestrogens from the soy milk that help even out any hormonal imbalances that might be dragging you down.

raspberries 3/4 cup

blackberries 2/3 cup

pomegranates 2, seeds and flesh scooped out

soy milk 1¼ cups, calcium-enriched

greek or plain whole milk yogurt 4 tablespoons

tahini 3 teaspoons

ancient wisdom

This is a United Nations of a smoothie, starting with the ancient wisdom of the Greeks (who still make real yogurt full of beneficial bacteria), and tahini, which is like peanut butter but made from sesame seeds. Next come pomegranates, with an ancient history in the Middle East; raspberries and blackberries, traditionally gathered wild in the hills of Scotland and the hedgerows of England; and soy products, which come to us from the Far East. They all combine to make you feel happier.

vital statistics

With brain-nourishing omega-3 fats from the tahini, improved production of B vitamins in the gut through the friendly bugs, mood-enhancing phytoestrogens from the soy milk, and all the protective nutrients in the berries and pomegranates, this has to be a double whammy of good mood and good health.

red grapes 1¹/₄ cups, seedless
pawpaw 2, seeded, flesh scooped out
kiwi fruit 3

clever kiwis

Yes, they are clever, those New Zealanders. Once they found out they could grow the Chinese gooseberry so successfully, they renamed it kiwi fruit. Juiced together here with grapes and pawpaw, this is a simple, nourishing, and good-mood drink.

vital statistics

The **natural enzymes** and **trace elements** in the pawpaw and kiwi fruit help to replace mood-sapping nutrient deficiencies. With the quick energy boost of the grapes as well as all their protective benefits, this is a great start to a lousy day.

pomegranates 2, seeds and flesh scooped out
granny smith apples 4
lime 1, peeled (unless key lime)
orange-blossom water 1 dash

middle eastern magic

The pomegranate, lime, and orange-blossom water are certainly Middle Eastern, but the Granny Smith apples are not. However, that doesn't stop this delicious bit of magic helping you enjoy a good mood for the rest of the day.

vital statistics

The **vitamin E** and **antioxidants** from the pomegranates and the small quantities of essential oils from the orange-blossom water all help to enhance your mood. The extra **vitamin C** from the apples and the lime will make sure you absorb sufficient iron from the food that follows this drink.

pears 2 large
celery 2 sticks, with leaves
chard (or sorrel leaves) 1 good handful, washed
mint 2 good sprigs
flaxseeds 2 teaspoons, ground

pear punch

Pears and celery normally go together with a strong piece of cheddar, but not here, because this juice packs a real punch, thanks to the flaxseeds.

vital statistics

Flaxseeds are the next best thing to fish oils in terms of omega-3 fatty acids and enhance mood and behavior. Mint, surprisingly, is not only the best antacid of all, but contains essential oils that sharpen concentration and focus, while the green leaves in this juice provide betacarotenes and small but important amounts of iron.

cucumber 1
apples 4
pineapple 1 small, peeled and sliced
flat-leaf parsley 1 medium bunch
basil 3 good sprigs
nonfat plain yogurt ½ cup
strawberries 2, hulled and quartered

the moody swinger

If the idea of strawberries, parsley, and basil sounds a bit strange, wait till you try them with balsamic vinegar and black pepper—a truly stunning taste combination. Using the other fruit and yogurt to produce this smoothie creates a unique taste that will give you a lot of pleasure and help lift your mood if you're feeling down in the dumps. Just put the first four ingredients and two sprigs of basil through a juicer, mix in the yogurt, and top with the strawberry quarters and remaining basil.

vital statistics

The aromatic esters from apples and the essential oils in basil are all calming and mood-enhancing. The cucumber and parsley have a gentle diuretic effect that helps with the fluid retention and swelling that some women get around their periods.

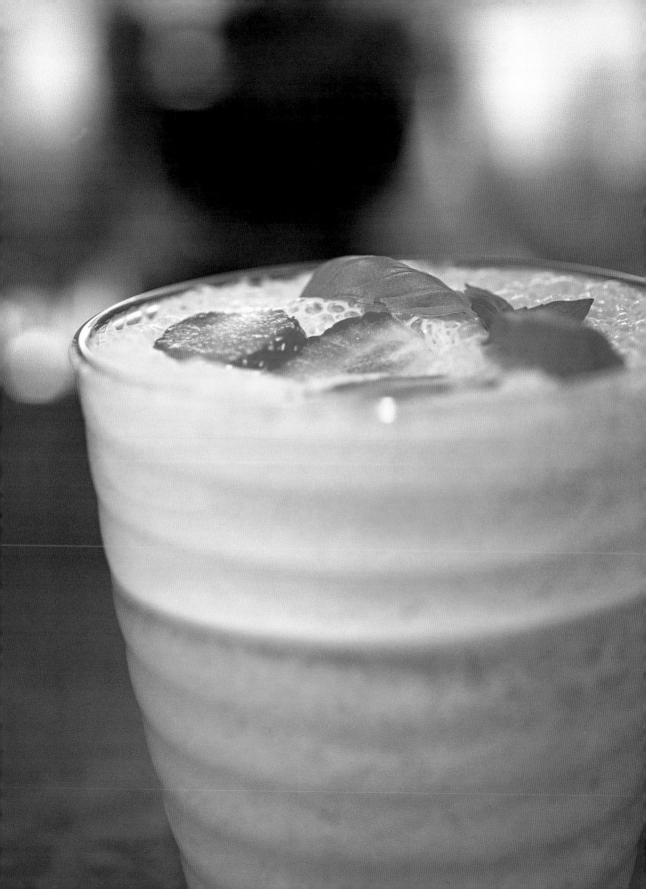

hot chocolate 3/4 mug, made from an organic, 70 percent cocoa solids mix

banana 1, ripe

honey 2 teaspoons

ground cinnamon 1 pinch

grated nutmeg 1 generous pinch

brainy bananas

You can't really get juice out of a banana but they're so nutritious that, combined in this juice, they make a real restorative drink to help you sleep, have sweet dreams, and ease any aching muscles if you've been boogieing the night away. Put it all in a blender and whiz. Enjoy while still warm.

vital statistics

This juice offers amazing mood-lifting **theobromines** in the chocolate; mild, good-mood hallucinogenic action from the nutmeg; and a feel-good factor of instant energy from the honey. Finally, there's slower-release energy from the banana, together with its mood-enhancing **vitamin B$_6$**.

celery 2 sticks, with leaves
english apples 3 good-sized (ideally Russets)
kiwi fruit 4
basil 6 good-sized leaves
grated nutmeg ½ teaspoon

bounce back

Once again, it's the mood-enhancing properties of basil and nutmeg and the calming effect of celery that help you bounce back from feeling miserable to being in a good mood.

vital statistics

Nutmeg contains a mild hallucinogen that certainly makes you feel good, and the essential oils in basil make it one of the most mood-enhancing of all the herbs. Juiced together with calming celery, energizing apples, and kiwi fruit, this is a real mood reviver at the end of a long, hard day.

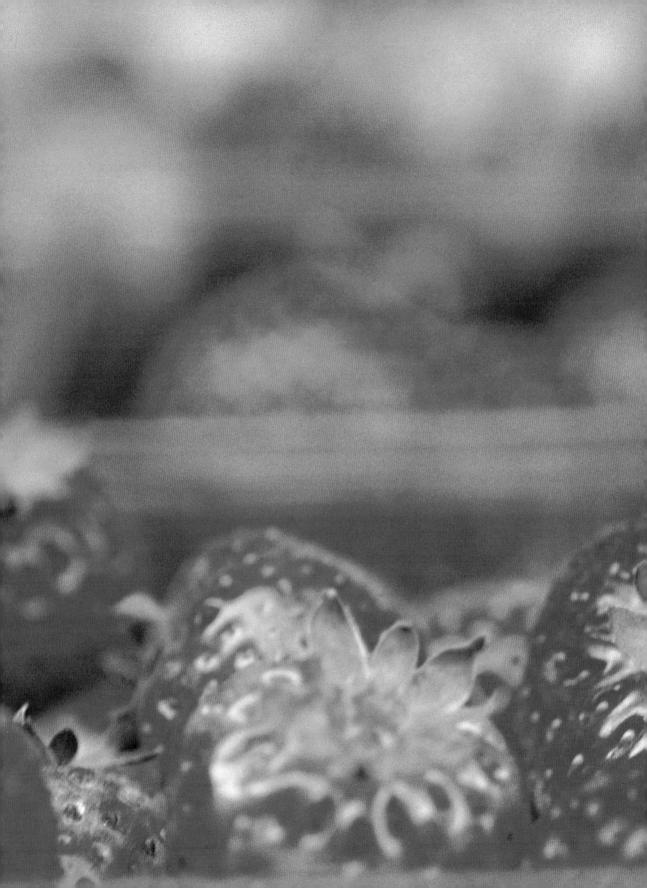

memory juices

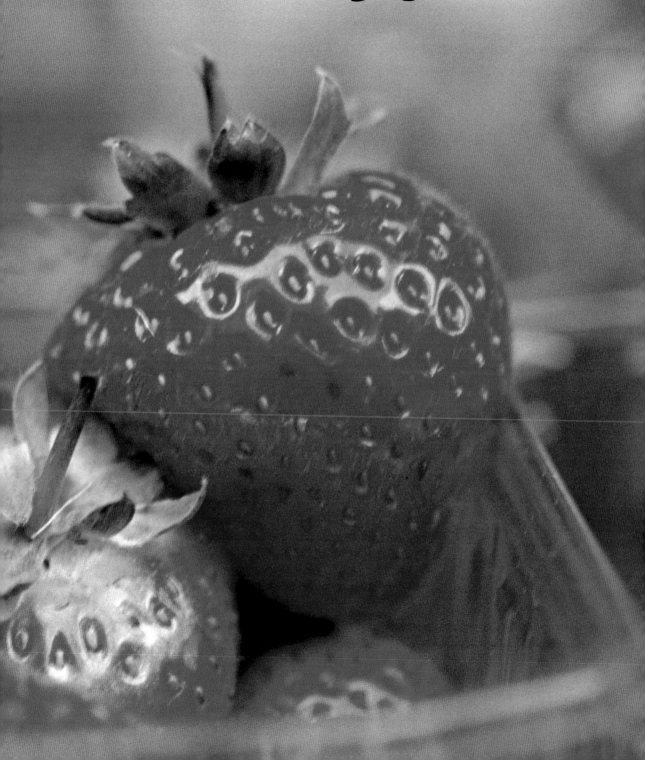

When your granny said "Eat your fish—it will make you brainy," she wasn't far off the mark. All oily fish contain essential fatty acids that make them vital foods for brain function. Fatty acids form a major part of the brain tissue, meaning these special fats are essential during pregnancy, breast-feeding, and childhood. But adults, too, need them to help maintain higher cognitive functions such as memory. Protein is also needed because it provides very slow-release energy that helps maintain the constant supply of blood sugar the brain needs to function efficiently. Non-animal sources of protein such as beans, lentils, and all the other legumes are also extremely valuable.

It's also important to limit your consumption of foods containing large amounts of saturated fat. One of the key factors in maintaining a good memory is doing everything you can to maintain the blood supply to the brain cells, and saturated fats can end up as fatty deposits inside the arteries, narrowing the size of the tubes, restricting blood flow, and adversely affecting memory and other brain functions. Vegetable proteins don't contain saturated fats, so they and organic poultry, game, and lean, free-range meat should be your first choices when it comes to reducing saturated-fat consumption.

The good news is that modest amounts of alcohol also help maintain good memory. The high levels of antioxidants that help protect the brain from local cell damage are found in abundance in red wine, so a couple of small glasses a day will do you good.

Herbs and spices have a vital role as brain foods as well. Some, such as basil, nutmeg, lemon balm, and cilantro, can affect mood and emotion, while others have a much more direct impact on your mental function. The most powerful of these are sage (synonymous with wisdom) and rosemary, which has been linked with improved memory since ancient times. Chili dilates the very smallest blood vessels, leading to an almost instant rush of blood to the head; this explains the beads of sweat on your forehead after your first mouthful of a strong chili sauce. Ginger also provides quick brain stimulation, whether you use fresh in juices or stir-fries, sprinkle powdered ginger on food and drinks, or take it as freshly made ginger tea.

Your brain is like the rest of your body: if you don't use it, you lose it. Keep it active by reading, doing puzzles, memorizing some poetry, and doing sums. Whether you write them down or use mental arithmetic, doing calculations is one of the most effective ways of maintaining a good memory.

melon 8 oz, yellow-fleshed, peeled and deseeded
kiwi fruit 2
cherries ½ cup, pitted
oranges the juice of 2
flaxseed oil 2 teaspoons

memories are made of this

Thanks to the essential fatty acids in the flaxseed, this unusual combination of flavors makes an effective memory, mood, and behavior tonic to add to your regular brain-boosting repertoire. Simply juice the melon, kiwi fruit, and cherries, add the juice of the oranges and the oil and stir well before drinking.

vital statistics

It's the omega-3 fatty acids from the flaxseed oil that really do the trick here. You can't really juice oily fish, and adding fish oils would make this unpalatable for most people. Flaxseed oil is virtually flavorless and odorless, so what you'll taste most is the unique flavor of cherries. Lots of vitamin C and even protective vitamin E from the seeds of the kiwi fruit will all add to the brain-boosting value.

yellow pears 4, very ripe
plums 4 sweet yellow
white grapes 1 bunch, seedless
lavender the flowers rubbed off of 2 stalks

peaceful pears

You may think it sounds odd to put lavender flowers in this delicious juice, but it isn't. It tastes and smells wonderful—and lavender has a direct effect on the brain. If you're having trouble sleeping this makes the perfect late evening drink. It also provides a huge boost in vitamin C which is important for good eyesight, and protection against everyday infections.

vital statistics

The **essential oils** in the lavender are extremely calming and sleep-inducing. They're also an excellent remedy for all types of headaches and enhance overall brain function. Combined with the **vitamin C** from the plums and pears and the large amount of **pectin** in the pears that protects against cholesterol deposits, you have an excellent brain boost, even without the natural sugars in the white grapes. These help maintain the essential sugar levels passing through the brain and add some antioxidant protection, too.

black grapes 3³/₄ cups, seedless

orange 1, peeled, but with pith

cloves 5

cinnamon 1 stick

nutmeg 1 generous grating

honey 1 tablespoon

mulled grape juice

Here's a delicious, warm and spicy drink that is not only enjoyable but also helps your memory. Juice the grapes, put the juice in a pan and add the orange juice and all the other ingredients. Warm through gently without boiling and strain before drinking.

vital statistics

The nutmeg, cinnamon, and cloves all have a beneficial effect on memory, mood, and brain function. The natural sugars in the grapes and honey help, too, plus you'll get a very large quantity of brain-protective antioxidants from the black grape skins.

plain yogurt 3/4 cup
skim milk 2/3 cup
chocolate powder 1 heaping tablespoon, organic,
plus 1 teaspoon for garnish
banana 1
ground nutmeg 1 sprinkle
ground cinnamon 1/2 teaspoon

aztec promise

Chocolate was discovered by the Aztecs, who considered it so valuable that only royal families consumed it. Known as the food of the gods, chocolate is renowned for its ability to improve mood and memory, and in this wonderful drink it combines the brain-feeding components of bananas with the mental stimulus of the tropical spices. The extra sting in the tail of this recipe is that it's a pretty good aphrodisiac, too. Process the first four ingredients in a blender, then top with extra chocolate, nutmeg, and cinnamon.

vital statistics

The gut-friendly bacteria in the yogurt produce **B vitamins** that are important for memory. The banana helps keep blood-sugar levels on an even keel: another vital factor in good brain function. Add the **theobromine** from chocolate, the mind-opening **myristicin** in nutmeg, and the **essential oils** from the cinnamon and you have a delicious mood-boosting, brain-enhancing, and memory-improving drink.

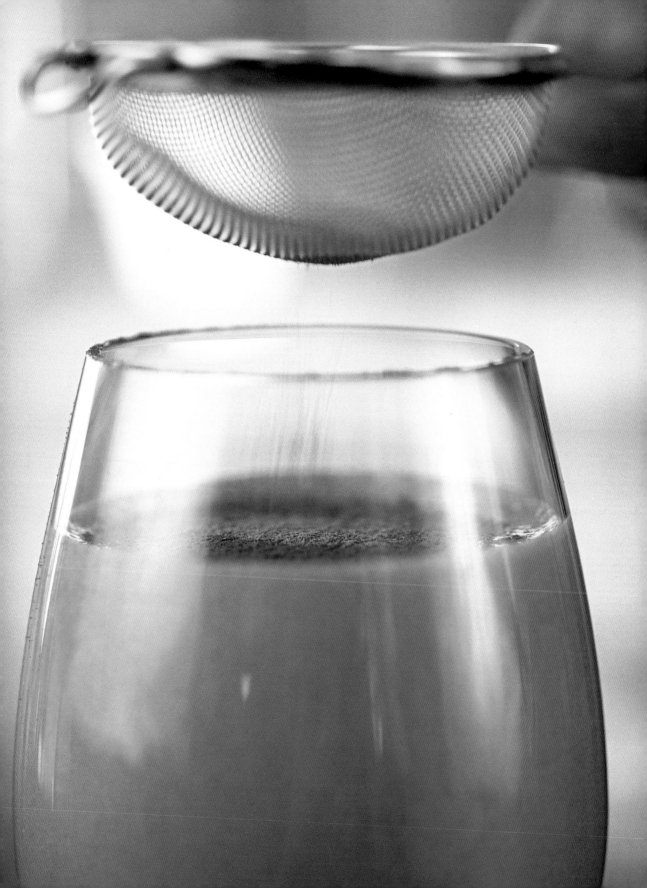

apples 3
pears 2
mango 1, peeled and pitted
strawberries 1⅓ cup, hulled
basil leaves 1 teaspoon

bedtime fruit salad

If you've had some studying to do during the evening and you want to make sure you remember it by morning, take a glass of this juiced fruit salad before you go to bed. You may think it sounds odd to add basil to these delicious fruits, but it's the aroma of this wonderful herb that gives the juice its unique flavor.

vital statistics

The memory boost comes from the **essential oils** in the basil, but it's enhanced by the **natural sugars** in the rest of the fruit and the brain-protective **antioxidants** in the strawberries. The large amount of **vitamin C** also helps the absorption of iron from your evening meal, reducing the risk of anemia. The soluble fiber **pectin** from the apples and pears increases the body's elimination of cholesterol and helps avoid artery-clogging deposits.

lychee 10, shelled and pitted

pomegranates 2, seeds and flesh scooped out

kumquats 2

guavas 2, peeled

grapefruit* 1, pink, peeled, but with pith

lucky lychee

Although widely available, not many people use kumquats, and even less use them in juices. Yet their bitter flavor in this brain-protective drink is masked by the sweetness of the other fruits and the unique taste of lychees: another fruit seldom used in juices but well worth the effort.

*If taking prescribed medicines, consult your doctor before drinking large amounts of grapefruit juice.

vital statistics

It's the natural red coloring that provides most of the protective antioxidants in this juice. The combined nutritional value of pomegranate, kumquats, and guavas is enhanced by the vitamin C from the grapefruit, which also serves as a brain-protective antioxidant.

kale 1 handful
garlic 2 cloves
parsley 1 handful
celery 1 stick, with leaves
carrots 2, topped and tailed, peeled if not organic
sweet potato 1 small

oracle juice

This juice is a good source of ORAC units (*see* page 142): the best way of measuring the total antioxidant protective value of whole foods. A glass of this juice will provide almost all you need for a whole day's protection. Taking your antioxidants in tablets does not work nearly as well as getting them from these high-ORAC foods.

vital statistics

The **essential oils** in parsley have a rapid and beneficial effect on the way your brain works. Add to this the juice of all the other ingredients and you'll get some **natural sugars**, lots of **betacarotene**, the diuretic effect of parsley, and the hugely cancer-fighting benefits of the kale. All this and memory, too!

butternut squash 1 lb, flesh only

carrot 1 large, topped and tailed, peeled if not organic

pomegranate 1, seeds and flesh scooped out

fresh rosemary 1 sprig finely chopped leaves

mineral water sparkling, to taste

sparkling squash

From the ancient Greeks and Romans onward, rosemary has been regarded as the herb of remembrance. Its natural constituents appear to act directly on the memory centers of the brain, and that's the building block of this interesting drink. Juice the squash, carrot, flesh of the pomegranate, and rosemary leaves and top up with sparkling mineral water to taste.

vital statistics

This drink provides an abundance of antioxidants that protect the brain and body from oxidative damage right down to the cellular level. It also provides an ideal medium to transport the rosemary into the digestive system, where its essential oils can be released to improve your memory.

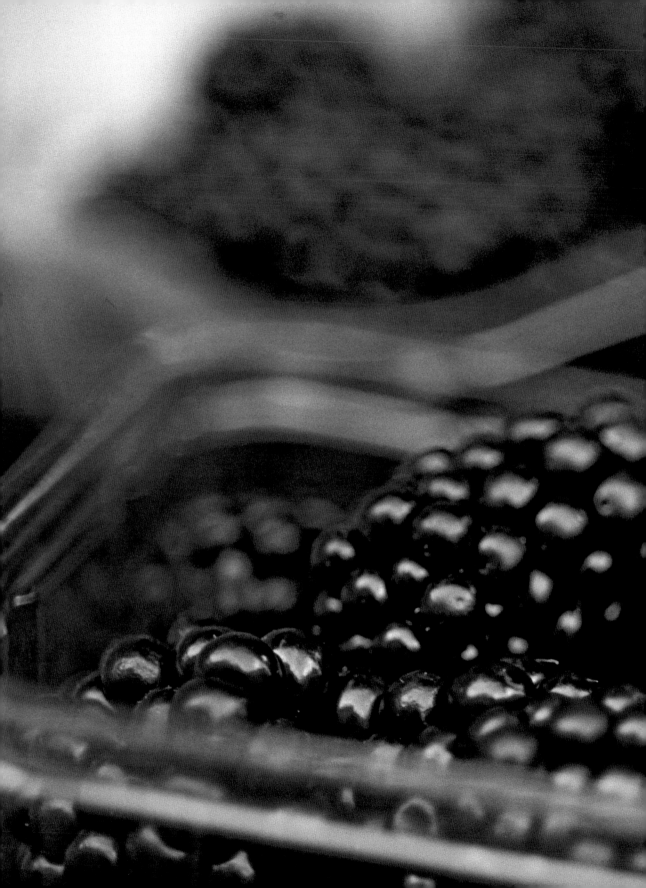

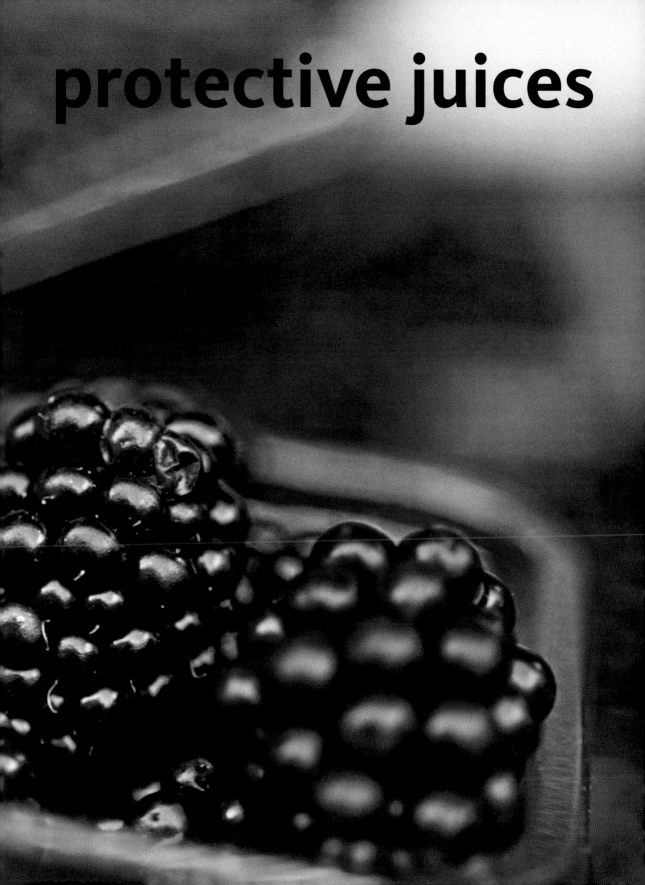

protective juices

There is no doubt that **widespread deficiency of nutrients plays a key role in people's diminishing natural immunity.** The obvious areas that need attention are vitamins and the macro-minerals; that is, those minerals such as iron, calcium and potassium needed in substantial quantities. Even the micro-minerals, which the human body needs in very small amounts, seem to be disappearing from our regular food intake—top of this list are zinc and selenium, with iodine a very close third.

But these are just the tip of the iceberg, because we need all the other nutrients that occur in food, too. Some of them we know about, such as betacarotene and essential fatty acids, but there are others we have only recently discovered, such as lutein and zeaxanthine, which are both essential to protect the eyes against age-related macular degeneration (AMD), the most common cause of poor sight and eventually blindness in older people.

We are also just discovering the importance of the cancer-fighting chemicals in plants such as cabbage, and scientists around the world are now studying this amazing family of vegetables. Some of the world's leading authorities on cancer, heart disease, strokes and degenerative diseases such as arthritis now believe that **the food chemicals we know about, possibly together with hundreds yet to be identified, play a major role in the body's ability to protect itself from disease.**

The whole antioxidant story is now unravelling to reinforce the importance of food. Interestingly, in studies that have been done using antioxidants such as vitamins A, C and E in isolation as supplements, the results have been disappointing and sometimes even negative. Yet repeat those same studies using food as the source of protective chemicals and the evidence of positive benefits is overwhelming. The juices in this chapter are rich sources of these protective nutrients.

strawberries 10 medium, hulled
kiwi fruit 2
passion fruit 2, flesh scooped out
blueberries 1 cup
pears 2
apples 1

a passion for fruit

Most fresh fruits are exceptionally rich sources of protective phytochemicals. The darker the color, the higher the ORAC score and their antioxidant protective properties. Strawberries have the additional benefit of helping to relieve the inflammation of inflammatory joint disease.

vital statistics

Kiwi fruits are uniquely rich in both vitamin C and vitamin E, both protective nutrients, and strawberries have an amazing ability to increase the body's elimination of uric acid, a substance that is highly irritating to inflamed joints in gout and arthritis. Second only to prunes, blueberries are, weight for weight, the next richest source of protective antioxidants.

cherries 1 cup, pitted
blueberries 2/3 cup
pears 2 large

cherry sunday

Cherries have been a favourite of herbalists for generations. You can use the bark of the tree, the stalks and even the stones for making remedies, but of course they are absolutely delicious to eat. Mixed here with the sweetness and perfume of really ripe pears, they make a protective juice that tastes excellent and will be enjoyed by children and adults alike. Removing the stones is a pain, but I promise it's worth the effort. Juice all the fruit and pour over ice for the perfect Sunday brunch immune-booster.

vital statistics

This recipe provides well over 4000 protective ORAC units (*see* page 142)—phenomenal considering 3500 ORACs is the recommended optimum consumption for a day. If you suffer any form of arthritis or gout, cherries help the body eliminate uric acid, one of the main causes of pain in these illnesses. Blueberries contain **phytochemicals** that help protect the eyes as well.

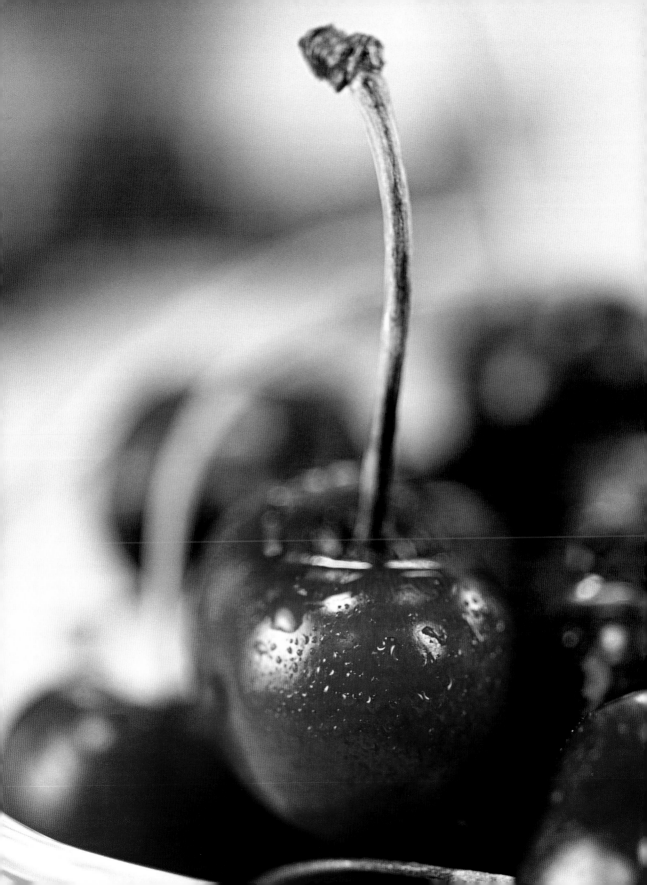

cranberries 2 cups, thawed if frozen
strawberries ⅔ cup
orange juice 6 tablespoons, freshly squeezed

cranberry source

Cranberries are an amazing fruit and were probably one reason why the early Pilgrims survived. Used by Native Americans for centuries as both food and medicine, they were introduced to the first settlers as the way of avoiding scurvy. They're not the sweetest of fruits, but combining them with strawberries and orange juice makes this a very refreshing drink.

vital statistics

Cranberries are an extremely rich source of **vitamin C**, but they have other even more important properties. They contain natural substances that prevent bacteria from attaching themselves to the walls of the bladder and urinary tract, which makes them both a treatment and a powerful preventer of cystitis and other recurring urinary infections.

black grapes 2¹/₂ cups, seedless
pears 2
limes 2, unpeeled unless key lime

sweet-and-sour power

People often think of pears as something you stick in the fruit bowl and probably throw away rotten before you've eaten them. What a mistake! Although they only contain small amounts of nutrients, they have other valuable properties and are the fruit least likely to cause any type of allergic reaction. In this highly protective sweet-and-sour juice, the sharpness of the limes complements the sweetness of the grapes and pears.

vital statistics

Pears contain no fat, virtually no sodium and a type of sugar easily converted into energy. With the heart-protective **phytochemicals** in the grapes and large quantities of **vitamin C** and **bioflavonoids** in the limes, this is a refreshing and unusual protective juice.

watermelon 2 lb, peeled, seeded
fresh gingerroot ½ inch, peeled
mango 1, peeled and pitted
coconut milk ½ cup

watermelon and coconut countdown

Watermelon makes the most refreshing of juices, but thanks to its wonderful red color it's also protective—even more so when combined with the stimulating effects of ginger and the rich nutritional value of mangoes. Juice the watermelon, gingerroot, and mango, then stir in the coconut milk.

vital statistics

Ginger contains a rich supply of **zingiberine,** which is a circulatory stimulant, speeding the blood flow and increasing the oxygenation of tissues, to help defend against free-radical damage. Mango is rich in natural **enzymes** and **betacarotenes,** and the watermelon provides **vitamin C.** The natural **fatty acids** in the coconut milk have anti-inflammatory properties.

sweet potato 1 large

baby spinach 2 handfuls, well washed

gingerroot 1 inch, peeled

black grapes 1 handful

apple 1

potato protector

Most people don't think about juicing sweet potatoes, but they do have a very pleasant and interesting flavor. You wouldn't want to drink it on its own, but with the spinach, ginger, and grapes it's not only palatable but helps protect the eyes, skin, and heart as well.

vital statistics

Sweet potatoes are an excellent source of betacarotene, and spinach provides the lutein and zeaxanthine, which protect eyes. When mixed with the circulation benefits of ginger, and the heart-protective action of the anthocyanins that color black grapes, this juice has many protective functions.

tomatoes 8, very ripe
gingerroot 1/2 inch, peeled
tabasco sauce 1 dash

hot tom

A healthier, more protective variation on canned tomato juice, this uses fresh tomatoes, stimulating ginger, and fiery Tabasco sauce. If you're feeling brave, add some vodka.

vital statistics

It's the combination of lycopene from the tomatoes, which protects against breast and prostate cancers, and the zingiberene from ginger and capsaicin in the Tabasco, both of which are circulatory stimulants, that add up to a delicious and highly protective drink.

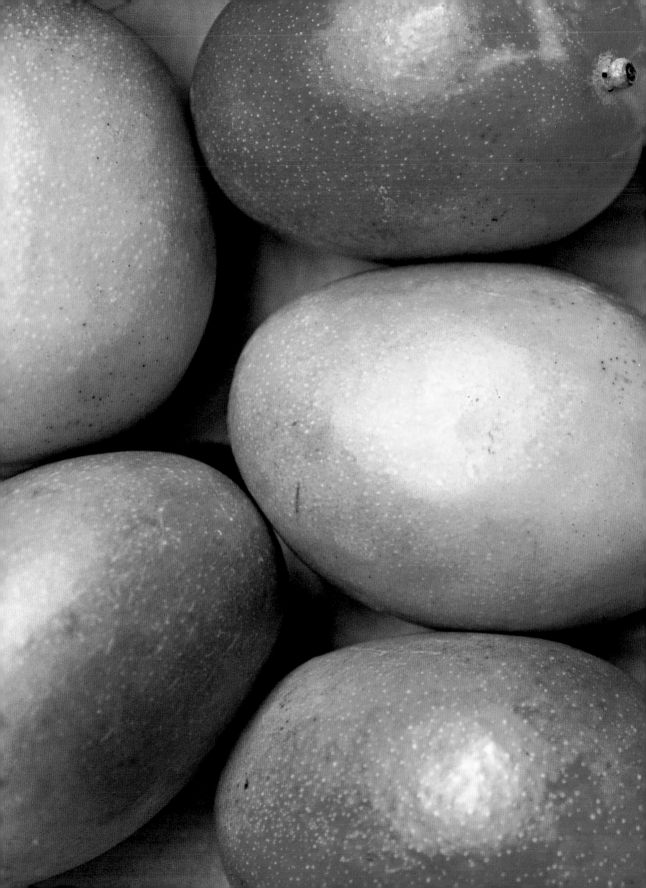

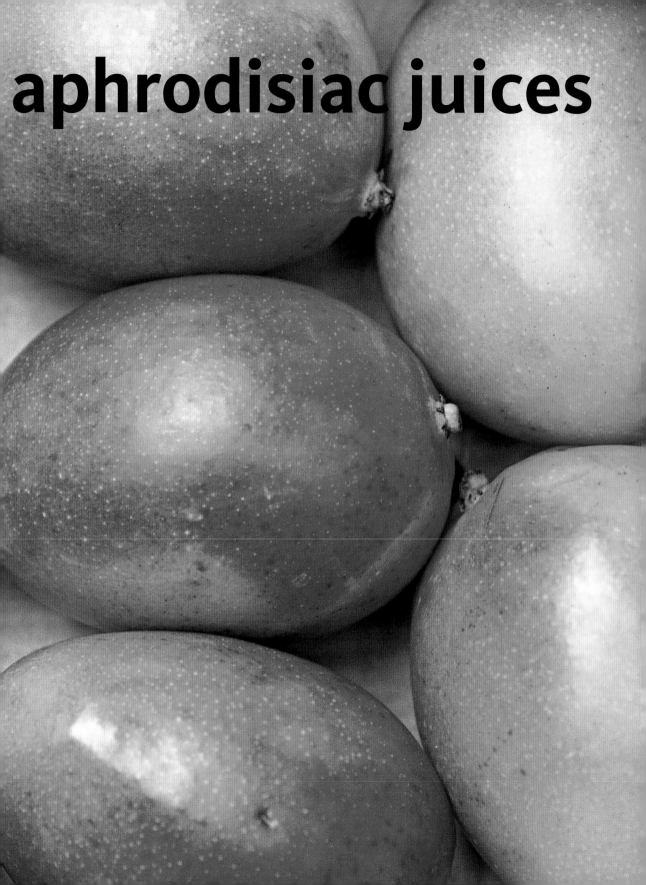

aphrodisiac juices

Living in the 21st-century poses a string of problems associated with desire, sex and conception. Until quite recently, most doctors considered male impotence to be predominantly a psychological problem, but how wrong they've been proved. Current opinion is now the reverse, since we now know that the plagues of diabetes, narrowed arteries and heart disease have a catastrophic effect on men's sexual ability. Add to this the fact that sperm counts have declined by around 50 per cent in the last 30 years and you get some idea of the scale of the problem.

Excessive consumption of saturated animal fats, a huge increase in the consumption of coffee and caffeinated drinks and too much alcohol are just part of the picture. Masses of refined carbohydrates and a world full of unwanted synthetic hormones from intensively reared animals and intensively produced dairy produce all add to the problem.

Strictly speaking, the only aphrodisiacs that work are either illegal or dangerous, but there's no doubt at all that some foods do lend a helping hand by igniting that flickering flame of desire that is all-important in a fulfilling relationship. In some parts of the Western world there's no avoiding the pressures of the 24/7 society, and this certainly can have a dramatic and disastrous effect on both male and female libido. If you couple this stressful lifestyle with poor nutrition, a satisfying sex life becomes even more unlikely.

A poor diet that contains too much of the artery-clogging, weight-gain-promoting and heart-disease-causing foods is just one side of the coin. The other side is a deficiency in the foods that provide vitamin E, zinc, selenium, iron, magnesium, and the other major nutrients that are essential for sex, fertility, conception and a healthy pregnancy.

These six aphrodisiac recipes are slightly tongue-in-cheek and without the backing of hard scientific evidence, but they are based on traditional folklore and all are a good source of the nutrients you need for good sexual health. They're certainly worth a try as they can't hurt. And you never know – they may help.

pomegranates 2, seeds and flesh scooped out

pawpaw 1, seeded, flesh scooped out

pears 3

apples 2 sweet such as Discovery

white grapes 1 cup, seedless

pomegranate power

The pomegranate, originally native to the Middle East, has been an ancient fertility symbol and traditional aphrodisiac because of its many seeds. It's regarded as a sacred mystical fruit in various parts of the world, but you won't know how good it is until you try it.

vital statistics

As well as the high content of vitamin E in the seeds of the pomegranate, the enzymes in the pawpaw, energy from the pears and the Bacchanalian image of grapes add to the aphrodisiac potential of this juice.

avocado 1 large organic Hass, pit and skin removed, cut into chunks

mango 1 large organic, peeled, pit removed, cut into chunks

beets 2 organic

goat milk 3/4 cup, organic

cilantro leaves 2 tablespoons

mangavo

Whether it's a lack of libido in either partner or male impotence that's causing a problem, there are foods that might help. Over the centuries, many things have acquired a reputation as aphrodisiacs and just knowing that can be enough to heighten sexual arousal. Avocados and mangoes both fall into this category. Used here with the mood-enhancing effects of cilantro, they'll help to put you in the mood. Juice the mango, beet and cilantro, then put in a blender with the avocado and goat milk.

vital statistics

The red coloring in the beet improves the oxygen-carrying capacity of blood, which in turn helps to boost the circulation—a prime requirement for male potency. Another essential nutrient is vitamin E, supplied by the avocado, while the mango contains betacarotene, some of which the body converts into vitamin A: an essential nutrient for the health and protection of mucous membranes.

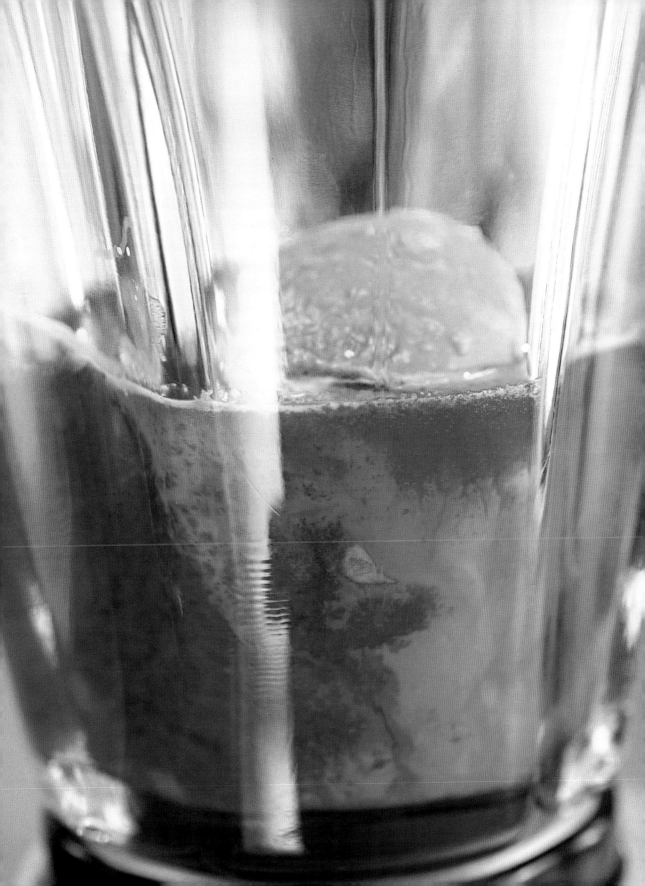

beets 3 medium
celeriac root 1/2
carrots 3 large, topped and tailed, peeled if not organic
cooking apple 1

beet bonanza

An extremely common cause of male impotence is poor blood supply to the penis. Anything that restricts the blood flow reduces a man's ability to have an erection and results in impotence. This juice may just help restore the confidence of any man who has had a problem.

vital statistics

The haemoglobin-like red coloring in beet helps increase the oxygen-carrying capacity of the blood; the large betacarotene content of carrots helps protect all the mucous membranes, including those of the urinary tract, and the high amount of pectin in the cooking apple helps reduce cholesterol, deposits of which in blood vessels can cause impotence.

radishes 6 large

carrots 4, topped and tailed, peeled if not organic

curly parsley 1 large handful, with stalks

swede a few chunks

radish rhapsody

You may be surprised at the thought that a chunk of swede, a handful of radishes and a few carrots could be aphrodisiac, but these are all sources of nutrients that are important for normal sexual function.

vital statistics

Like cabbage, broccoli and sprouts, radishes are a member of the *Cruciferae* family and are protective against cancer. They're also rich in potassium, calcium, vitamin C and selenium, a mineral that is universally deficient in most Western diets and vital for sexuality.

turnip 1 small, with top
beets 2 small, with leaves
parsnip 1 medium
sweet potato 1 small
carrots 2, topped and tailed, peeled if not organic

raunchy roots

Another strange-sounding mixture that most people would not associate with all-consuming passion (it really tastes much, much nicer than it sounds). Thanks to the root vegetables, it's a cornucopia of nutrients needed for sex, and if you love root vegetables, then this is just the one for you.

vital statistics

Sweet potatoes are a great source of complex carbohydrates—and therefore of energy. They provide a huge quantity of different carotenoids, and it's these and the other phytochemicals that make them an exceptional cancer-fighting food, especially if you're a smoker. It's the trace minerals in all the root vegetables that make them so useful as potential aphrodisiacs.

asparagus 4 spears

carrots 3, topped and tailed, peeled if not organic

chard 1 handful of leaves

bok choy 2 heads

pumpkin seeds 2 teaspoons

love in a glass

Asparagus is one of the traditional aphrodisiac foods. It has been used for medical purposes for at least 500 years and cultivated as a vegetable for more than 2000. This is a vegetable that really does need to be eaten in season if you're going to enjoy its maximum flavor and benefits. In this juice you can't detract from its health benefits by smothering it in butter, mayonnaise, hollandaise sauce, or piles of grated cheese.

vital statistics

A natural plant chemical called asparagine gives asparagus its diuretic effect and the unmistakable smell of your urine after eating it. It's great if you've got rheumatism or arthritis, but avoid it like the plague if you have gout. Pumpkin seeds add vital zinc, often lacking and essential not only for the health of the prostate gland but also for male sexuality. Chard and bok choy provide small amounts of iron, that help guard against anemia, another cause of impotence.

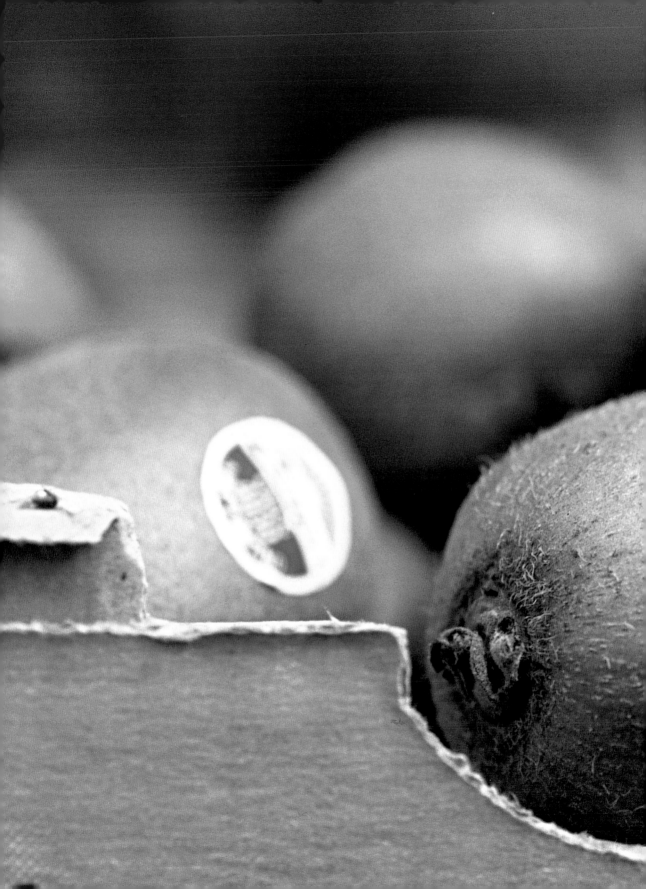

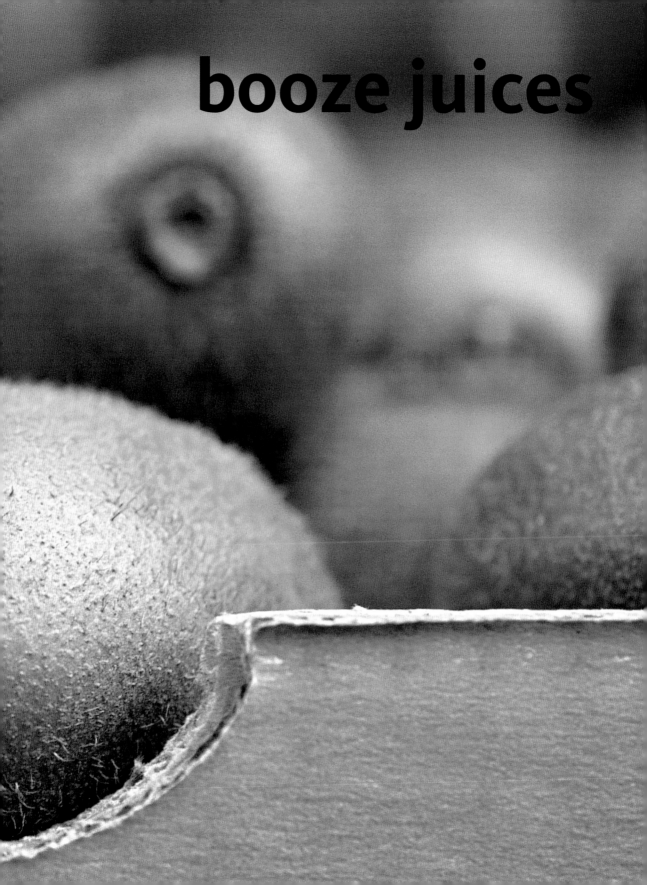

booze juices

What can I say? The recipes in this chapter are all juices with added booze—and there's nothing wrong with that, as long as you keep the alcohol within sensible proportions. From a health point of view, my advice is that women should stick to no more than 14 alcohol units a week and men should drink no more than 21. One unit of alcohol is the equivalent of 1.5 oz of spirits, a modest-sized glass of wine, or a 12 oz bottle of normal-strength beer, lager, or cider.

Saving all your units up for a binge on Friday night is bad news for your liver, and for those who are fairly serious social drinkers these quantities may seem ridiculous. Unfortunately, alcohol-related liver disease and alcoholism are increasing at a rapid rate, especially among young women, whose alcohol tolerance is lower than a man's. The recommended units represent the amount of alcohol the experts believe to be the maximum safe average that avoids the risk of alcohol-related disease.

There is no doubt that small amounts of alcohol taken on a regular basis can actually be a health bonus. Red wine, for instance, is known to contain powerful protective anti-oxidants from the natural colorings in grape skins. Even spirits can have a positive effect on blood flow, blood pressure and heart health if consumed in small quantities. The truth is that statistically very moderate social drinkers have a slightly longer life expectancy than total abstainers. Cynics might say that many abstainers are recovering alcoholics in whom the damage has already been done, but many of the long term studies have been performed on social and religious groups for whom alcohol is forbidden. There is, however, absolutely no doubt that people who consistently drink large amounts of alcohol have the shortest life expectancy of all three groups.

It's a common misconception that alcohol is a stimulant because it makes you feel good, but the exact opposite is true. You feel good because alcohol depresses the inhibitory centers of the brain making you feel more extrovert, and the modest amounts in all these recipes are enough to have this pleasant effect, without the dreadful depression that follows a booze binge. These drinks also have the benefit of the added nutritional value from the other fresh ingredients. So do enjoy them—but enjoy them in moderation

strawberries 3 cups, hulled
pears 2 sweet
lime juice of 1
superfine sugar for coating
pink champagne 1 bottle

perry with a difference

This drink is guaranteed to lift the spirits, improve the mood, and blow away the clouds of depression. Also, it makes eight glasses, so get your friends round to share in the festivities! To make it, thoroughly chill the fruit and Champagne. Squeeze the lime, dip the rim of each Champagne flute into the juice, then into the superfine sugar and refrigerate the glasses. Juice the fruit, half-fill each glass, and top carefully with the Champagne.

vital statistics

Small amounts of alcohol are a gentle stimulant, but more is not better. Larger amounts cause depression—which will leave you crying into your glass if you overdo it.

peaches 3 large pink
pomegranate 1, seeds and flesh scooped out
pink champagne ½ bottle, iced

a better bellini

Nothing gives you a lift as quickly as a glass of good bubbly, and if you want to add a bit of great nutritional health, too, just add this fruit. The traditional Bellini uses only peaches, but by adding the pomegranate, the flavor just bursts out of the glass—and the color is astounding. This recipe will serve two. Simply juice the peaches and the scooped out flesh and seeds of the pomegranate, pour into chilled Champagne flutes, and top with Champagne.

vital statistics

The two glasses of alcohol you each get from half a bottle of Champagne is the safe and beneficial amount for a day, but adding the fruit provides **betacarotene**, **vitamin C**, and a selection of heart-protective and cancer-preventing nutrients.

pawpaw 1, seeded, flesh scooped out

mangosteen 1, cut in half, flesh scooped out

guavas 2, peeled

plain yogurt 1/2 cup

coconut milk 1 cup

crushed ice plenty

malibu 2 measures

grated nutmeg to taste

on the beach

Just the smell of coconut will transport you to the tropical isles, and the gentle kick of Malibu will help you on the way. Juice all the fruit, put into a blender with the yogurt, coconut milk, crushed ice, and Malibu, pour into two chilled highball glasses, sprinkle with the nutmeg and enjoy. (Paper umbrellas and sunglasses optional.)

vital statistics

You'll get masses of **bioflavonoids** for skin, eyes, mucous membranes and natural resistance. The essential **fatty acids** in the coconut milk and the feel-good factor of the mild hallucinogens in nutmeg are an added bonus. Put your deck-chair by the window and the rain clouds and thunder will soon turn into a tropical sky and rolling surf breaking on the golden beach—well, we can all dream...

apples 4 mild-flavored (like Golden Delicious)
sweet potato 1 small
carrot 1, topped and tailed, peeled if not organic
fresh mint 2 sprigs
jack daniel's whiskey 2 measures

applejack

As a cooling nightcap on a hot summer's evening, nothing could be finer in the state of Carolina—or anywhere else for that matter. Wash the fruit and vegetables, juice them and pour over ice into highball glasses. Add a measure of whiskey to each and insert a sprig of mint.

vital statistics

This small amount of alcohol is a heart stimulant, improves the circulation, and helps protect against heart disease, strokes, and narrowing of the arteries. The soluble fiber in the apples helps reduce cholesterol, and the betacarotene in the carrot and sweet potato is good for the skin and immune system. The mint oil which dissolves into the alcohol is an excellent digestive, either before or after a meal.

carrots 2, topped and tailed, peeled if not organic
bok choy 2 heads
mixed chinese greens 1 large handful
scallions 2
bean sprouts 1 handful
white radish 1 large
fresh gingerroot 1 inch
sake (Japanese rice wine) 2 measures

stir-fry cocktail

This is kitchen medicine at its best, used for prevention rather than cure. Wash and juice all the vegetables. Warm the juice slightly, mix with warmed rice wine, and enjoy with a meal.

vital statistics

This is another high-ORAC (*see* page 142) drink with powerful protective elements in all the vegetables. Anti-cancer, anti-diabetes, and immune-boosting ingredients make this a genuine super juice for all-round protection and good health.

beets 2, with leaves
turnips 2 small, with leaves
apples 2
carrots 3
vodka to taste

siberian sling

As the name implies, this booze juice is perfect for the coldest winter day. Beets, turnips, and carrots are typical Russian winter vegetables as they all store well through the biting cold months on the Siberian plains. Even with the vodka, this is a seriously healthy drink to boost your circulation—just don't exceed two 1.5 oz measures a day to stay within the maximum safe alcohol consumption for both men and women.

vital statistics

You'll get blood-building nutrients from the beet, all the cancer-protective phytochemicals from turnips, masses of betacarotene from the carrots, with vitamin C and pectin from the apples. So this is a protective, energizing and immune-boosting shot in the arm.

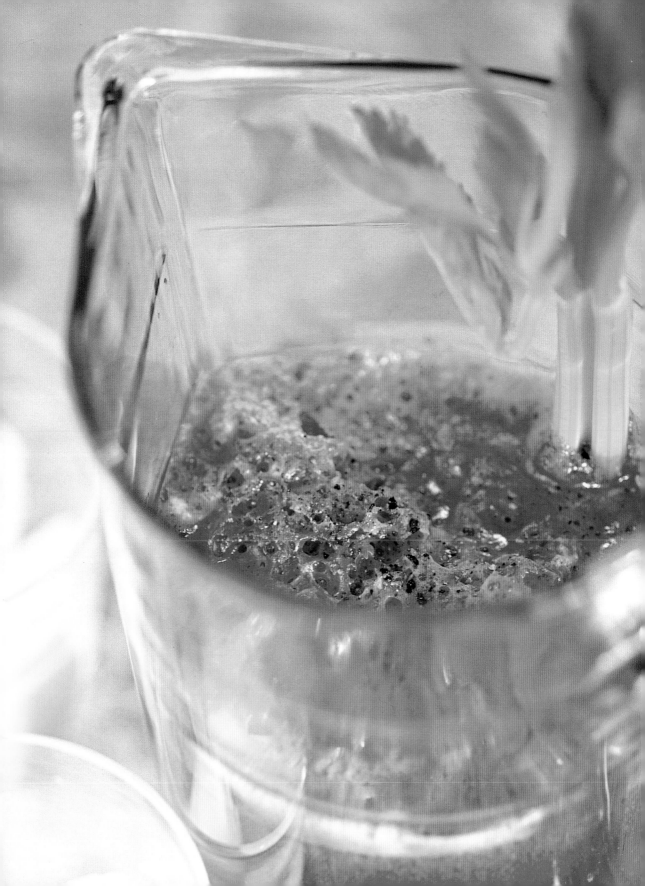

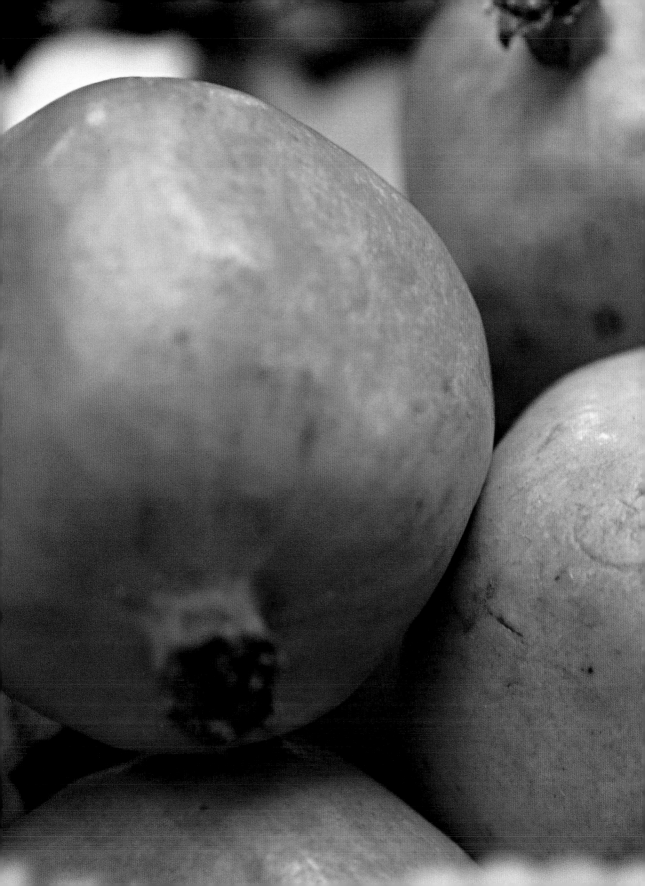

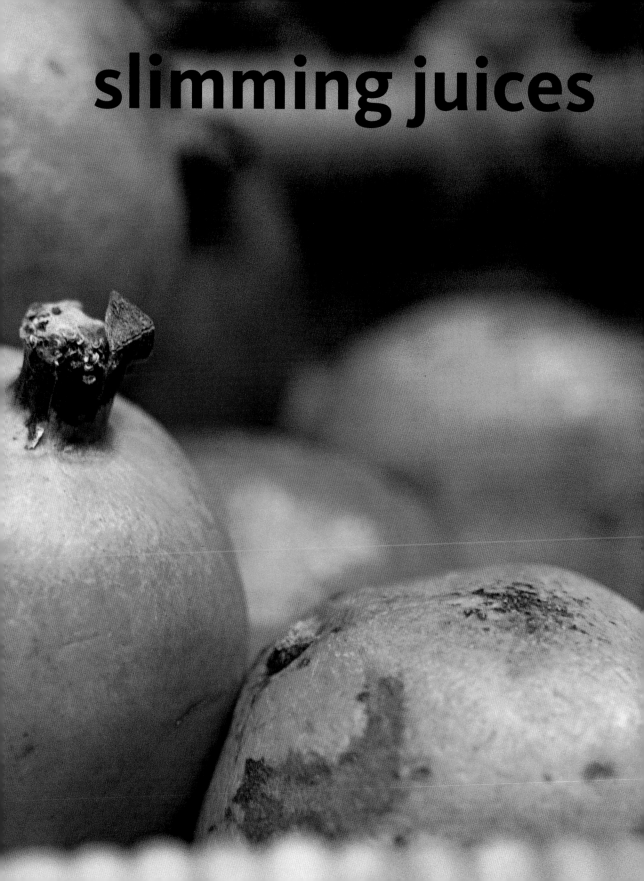

slimming juices

There are no juices that will make you thin unless you also reduce your total calorie consumption. Having said that, the juices in this section will help as part of a sensible, calorie-controlled diet. Some will help you get rid of fluid. Some, like A Prickly Customer (*see* page 109), help control appetite and reduce the hunger pangs, while others help you feel good and overcome the misery of trying to stick to a diet. The simple truth is that diets don't work. Although you may be able to lose 10 lbs in 10 days, you'll put back 12 lbs in the next 7 days once you go back to eating normally. Meal replacements, special drinks and weight loss pills are also best avoided.

The only thing that does produce long-term benefits is changing the way you eat so that you're enjoying your food and making the right choices, without sticking to some rigid, boring, and frustrating eating plan that makes you weigh and measure everything you put in your mouth. The perfect way to control your weight is a combination of sensible eating and moderate exercise, as this avoids the excesses of very low-calorie diets, or extreme exercise programmes, both of which can be harmful. For normal everyday purposes the minimum calorie requirement is 1500 a day for women and 2000 for men—if you consume less than this, you won't be eating enough essential nutrients. The trick is to eat a few less calories, and to burn a few more, for example, by eating two slices of bread and butter a day less, and walking briskly for 15 minutes a day more you will lose around 1 lb a week.

All of these eight slimming juices provide healthy nutrients and interesting flavors. But you can't live on them alone—and you shouldn't have more than two glasses a day.

watercress 2 handfuls
flat-leaf parsley 2 handfuls
cantaloupe melon 1, peeled, seeded and sliced
mango 1, peeled, pit removed
lime the juice of 1

waterfall 2

Flat-leaf parsley's richer, fuller and slightly smoother flavor makes it a more appealing ingredient here than the English curly variety. However, its use in this juice is mainly as a diuretic to help ease stubborn fluid retention. To make Waterfall 2, thoroughly wash the watercress and parsley and roll into cigar shapes. Feed these into the juicer between the melon and mango. Squeeze and strain the lime juice, then add to the mixture and stir.

vital statistics

As stated above, parsley is a gentle diuretic that helps remove excess body fluid. Watercress is rich in iron and cancer-fighting chemicals and is an energizing vegetable if you're restricting your food intake. Melon and mango provide an instant energy lift to keep you going till the next meal.

prickly pear 1
pomegranates 2, seeds and flesh scooped out
passion fruit 3, flesh scooped out

the three ps

This juice is a combination of three fairly strange fruits, some of which you may never have eaten. Pomegranates and passion fruit taste fabulous, but it's the prickly pear that makes this juice an effective aid to weight loss. Many supermarkets now stock all these fruits, but if you have any difficulties you'll often find them in Middle Eastern and Asian speciality food stores. Simply juice the flesh and seeds from the pomegranates and passion fruit with the prickly pear.

vital statistics

Widely eaten throughout Mexico and other parts of South America, where the flesh of both the fruits and leaves are consumed, prickly pears have the ability to curb the appetite, slow digestion, and minimize the feelings of hunger. Put this together with the high **natural sugar** content of pomegranates and passion fruit and you get a combination of instant and slow-release energy which is the ideal mid-morning, mid-afternoon, or mid-evening drink to prevent that diving blood-sugar level between meals—so often the trigger for binge eating on high-sugar, high-fat foods.

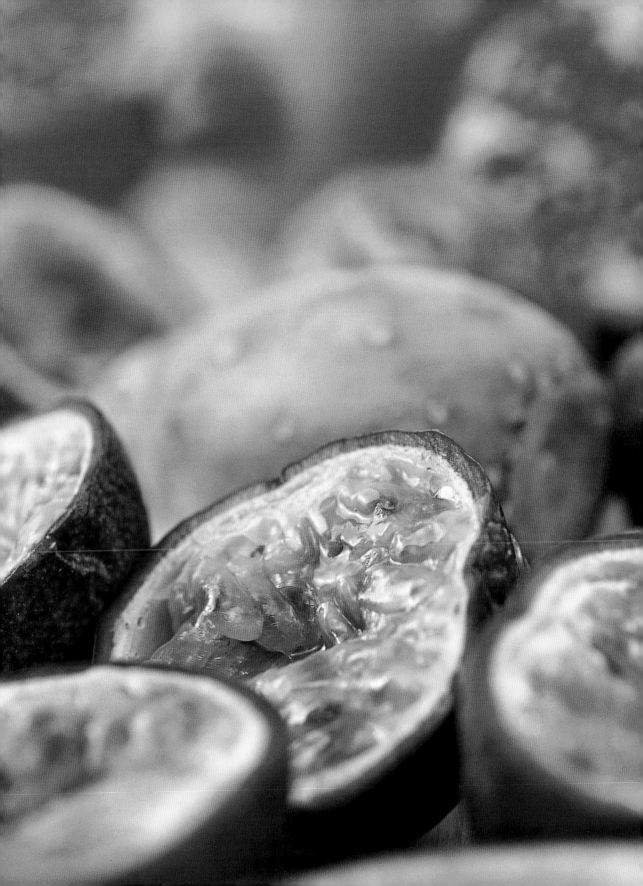

kumquats 4
key limes 2
green limes 2, peeled
pink grapefruit* 1, peeled, but with pith
blood oranges 2, peeled, but with pith
pomelo or ugli fruit 1, peeled

citrus slimmer

The pomelo is the early ancestor of the grapefruit and originates from Malaysia. Although the rind is thick, it's easy to peel, and the fruit has a wonderful sweet, spicy tang. If you can't find one, use an ugli fruit; these fruits were originally found growing wild in Jamaica back in the 1920s; the fresh, clean flavor is delicious. Kumquats and key limes will go through a juicer without any special preparation. Then, just mix their juice with that of the other fruit, which should be juiced by hand or with a citrus juicer. This drink is packed with nutrients for those on a diet.

*If taking prescribed medicines, consult your doctor before drinking large amounts of grapefruit juice.

vital statistics

The enormous amount of vitamin C will help boost the immune system while you're on a restricted diet, and the essential oils in the citrus fruits are an ideal cleanser to use during any detox regime. An additional bonus is the large quantity of protective bioflavonoids in the pith of all citrus fruits.

prickly pears 2
watermelon 3 thick slices, peeled and seeded
kiwi fruit 2

a prickly customer

You may never have bought or used this fruit of the prickly pear cactus, which, until recently, was mostly available in speciality ethnic food stores. Now even supermarkets stock this native Mexican fruit. It can also be found growing in parts of the Mediterranean. This juice is great for reducing hunger pangs.

vital statistics

The prickly pear's value is as an aid to weight loss, thanks to its ability to reduce sensations of hunger. It has a similar aroma to watermelon but a far more intense flavor.

apricots 6, pitted
pineapple ½ small, peeled
carrots 2 large, topped and tailed, peeled if not organic
grated nutmeg to taste

nutmeg nectar

This is a filling and sustaining juice that provides both a short- and long-term energy release to keep you going between your diet meals. Juice all the produce, pour over ice cubes and sprinkle with fresh grated nutmeg.

vital statistics

Adding the nutmeg provides a genuine feel-good factor that helps prevent the inevitable miseries of following a restricted-food weight-loss plan.

cucumber 1/2
little gem lettuce 1
dandelion 1 good handful of leaves
apples 2 green such as Granny Smiths
scallions 2 whole
watercress 1 handful

pis en lit

In the north of England, the country name for dandelion is "wet the bed." In France, it's *pis en lit*. This green juice lives up to its name in either country—not, I hasten to add, literally—but it is an effective diuretic, with all the additional health benefits of watercress and apples.

vital statistics

As well as helping you eliminate fluid, this juice is also a blood-building tonic that keeps you going when you're trying to reduce your food intake.

beets 2 medium, with leaves

celery 3 sticks, with leaves

pear 1 large

carrot 1, topped and tailed, peeled if not organic

spinach 1 handful, well washed

stop gap

If you're trying to lose weight, have a glass of this juice at least every other day—it's good for both brain and brawn. The beets helps maintain healthy blood and stops you feeling tired, and the fiber from the other ingredients makes this a thick and filling juice which controls sensations of hunger—making it easier for you to resist temptation.

vital statistics

One of the problems with any weight-loss regime is between-meal snacking. Whether it's hunger or habit, it's always hard to resist, but this juice is the perfect stop gap. Low in calories, rich in instantly available energy from the natural sugars in the beets, it will help you through the difficult times.

jerusalem artichokes 4
fennel 1 small bulb, with leaves
tomatoes 3 large
pears 3

prebiotic bonus

There's a growing interest in the role of probiotics (gut-friendly bacteria) as a general promoter of good digestion and improved natural resistance. Yet it's no good having the good bugs if they can't survive due to lack of the special food that they need. These particular nutrients, called prebiotics, are found in the unique form of fiber in the artichokes and pears in this recipe.

vital statistics

Getting enough of the **prebiotics** makes sure that the probiotics can do their job and encourage better digestion of nutrients. This juice will help make sure that all the **nutrients** you need can be extracted from food and absorbed during digestion.

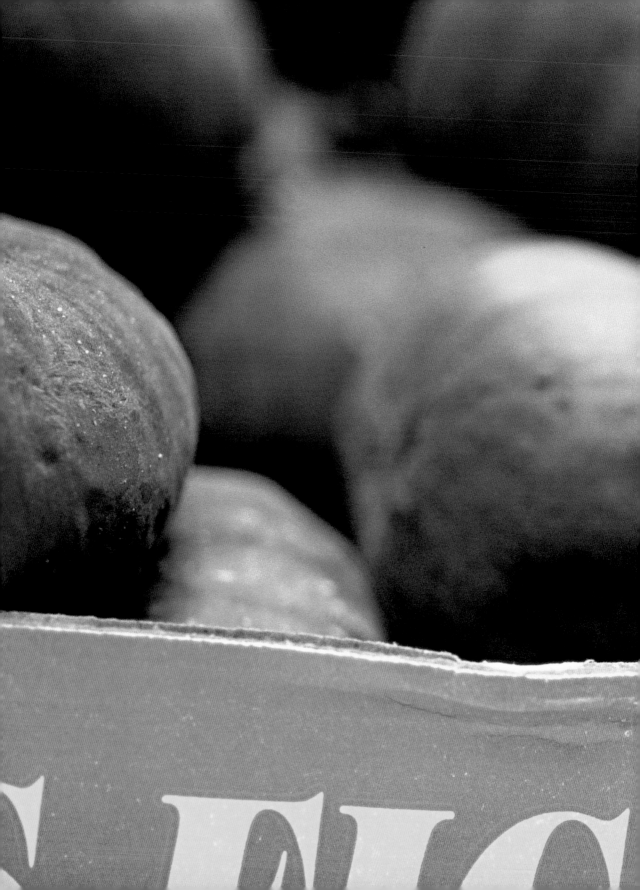

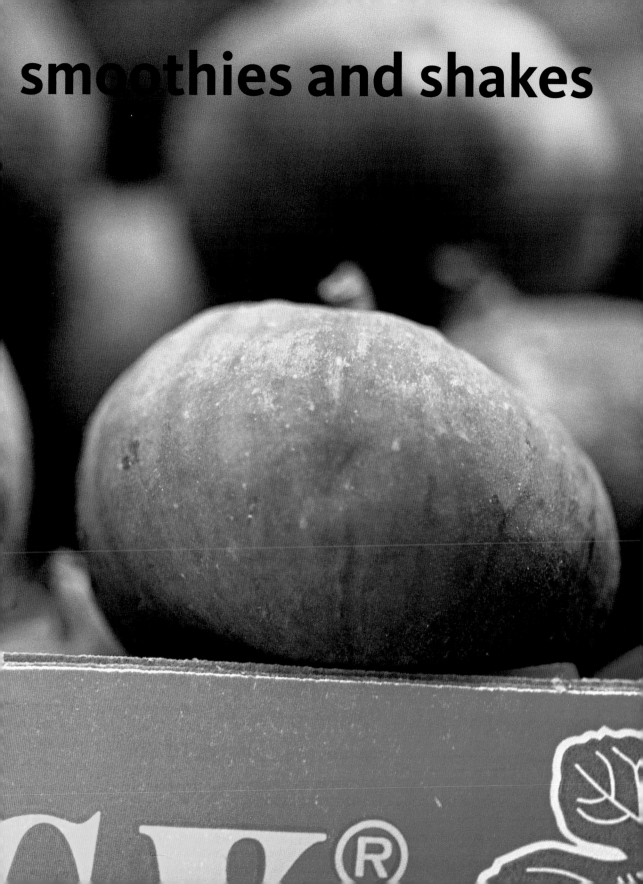

smoothies and shakes

soy milk 2 cups, calcium-enriched

sheep milk or plain yogurt 2/3 cup

banana 1

dried apricots 4, ready to eat

smooth peanut butter 3 tablespoons

ground walnuts 2 teaspoons

maple syrup 2 teaspoons

wheatgerm 2 teaspoons

brewer's yeast powder 2 teaspoons

liquid muscle

Place all the ingredients in a blender and whiz until smooth. Drink half in the morning, refrigerate the rest and drink it later in the day. It's an interesting flavor, but if you really don't like it, add a dessertspoon of good-quality dark chocolate powder.

vital statistics

This is the ideal drink for those trying to put on weight as it provides a terrific combination of quick- and slow-release energy with muscle-building **protein** but very little saturated fat. It's a good choice for athletes, too, and should be taken an hour before sporting activities for energy and stamina and an hour or two afterward to replace lost nutrients.

cranberries 1/2 cup, thawed if previously frozen

black currants 1/2 cup

blueberries 1 1/3 cups

dried apricots 2, ready to eat

dried prunes 2, ready to eat

plain yogurt 2/3 cup

whole milk 2/3 cup

cranberry jelly 2 teaspoons

flaxseed oil 2 teaspoons

beat the bugs

This is the ideal smoothie for youngsters starting school, where they're exposed to many new bugs; it's also ideal for all of us during times when colds and flu are spreading like wildfire. Put all the ingredients in a blender and whizz until smooth. The antibacterial activity of the cranberries, black currants, and plain yogurt all help boost the body's natural immune defences.

vital statistics

The exceptionally high ORAC score (see page 142) of this smoothie adds up to well over the optimum protective level and helps boost the body's resistance to viral, bacterial, or fungal attack.

strawberries 1½ cups, hulled
orange juice 3/4 cup, freshly squeezed
orange zest 2 teaspoons
superfine sugar 1 teaspoon
cottage cheese 1 cup
granola 1 cup organic, sugar-free

strawberry sundae smoothie

Put all the ingredients except the granola into a blender and whiz until smooth. Add the granola, stir, and serve sprinkled with the orange zest. This is best eaten with a spoon rather than drunk, even though it really is a smoothie.

vital statistics

Contains plenty of high-fiber and low-GI carbohydrates, a good dose of vitamin C, and all the beneficial nutrients in the strawberries.

blueberries 2 cups
ricotta ½ cup
milk ½ cup, low-fat

blueberry fool

This smoothie is really a cheesecake but without the cake—that's what makes it healthy. Put the blueberries and ricotta into a blender and whiz until smooth. Thin with milk to the desired consistency.

vital statistics

The **antioxidant** protection that cares for every cell in your body comes from the blueberries, with lots of other nutrients from the milk and ricotta cheese, turning this extremely delicious, quick, and simple recipe into a potent healing potion.

pineapple 1 small, peeled
mango 1 medium, peeled, without pit
bananas 2
coconut milk 1 x 14 fl oz can

tropical sport

What could be more tropical than these wonderful fruits? This is perfect an hour before or straight after any sort of sporting endeavor, but who needs an excuse? Tropical Sport is a great smoothie for adults and kids alike, as it is full of vitality, satisfying, and easily digested. Add it to the diet of those trying to gain weight, or use as a meal substitute if you are dieting. Peel and juice the pineapple and mango, then blend with the banana and coconut milk.

vital statistics

Healing **enzymes** in the pineapple and mango as well as lots of instant energy from their **fruit sugars**, plus the slow-release calories, **potassium** and **vitamin B$_6$** in the bananas are what provide the healing benefits.

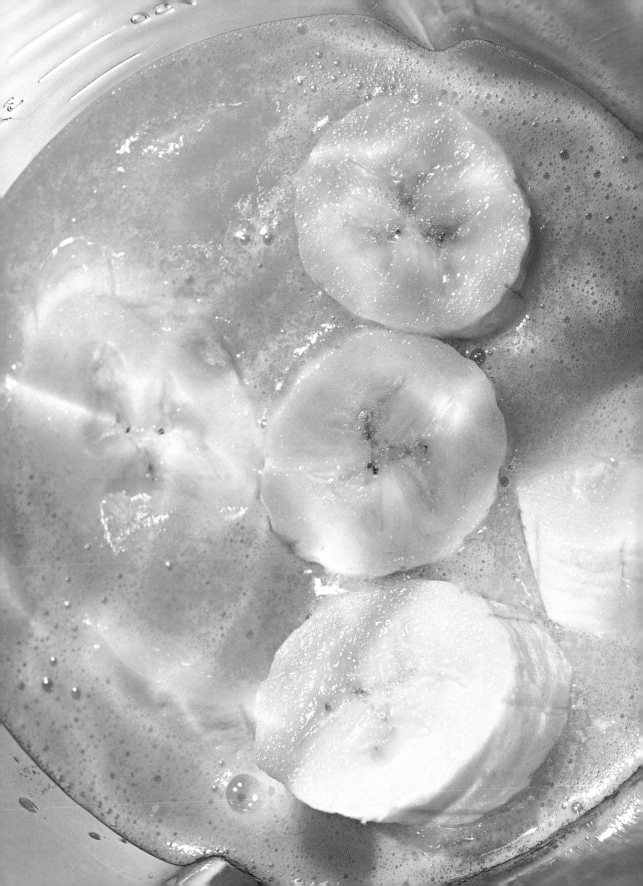

soy milk 1¼ cups, calcium-enriched

tofu 7 oz

cantaloupe melon ½ small, peeled, seeded and chopped

ogen melon ½ small, peeled, seeded and chopped

honeydew melon ½, peeled, seeded and chopped

honey 1 tablespoon

ice cubes 1 handful

boney m

Although osteoporosis is much more common in women, it does affect men too, so here's a drink that's good for everyone at any age. It's an interesting combination and a superb bone-builder. Simply put all the ingredients into a blender and whiz.

vital statistics

This juice is ideal for women as it has the added advantage of all the natural plant hormones in the tofu and soy milk, which help with PMS and menopausal symptoms. Of course there's also the added benefit of nutrients from the melons.

apples 2
figs 2
apricots 4 fresh
low-fat plain yogurt 1¼ cups
greek honey 1 tablespoon
pine nuts 3 tablespoons, toasted

a smooth greek

Juice the apples, figs, and apricots and combine with the honey and yogurt. Sprinkle with the toasted pine nuts—simply put the nuts into a preheated dry skillet and keep shaking over a high heat until they start to brown and crisp.

vital statistics

This traditional Greek combination of yogurt, pine nuts, and honey is a great source of calcium, protein, and energy. When made into a smoothie with the apple, fig, and apricot juice, you end up with a delicious and highly nutritious combination that looks good and tastes better than you can possibly imagine.

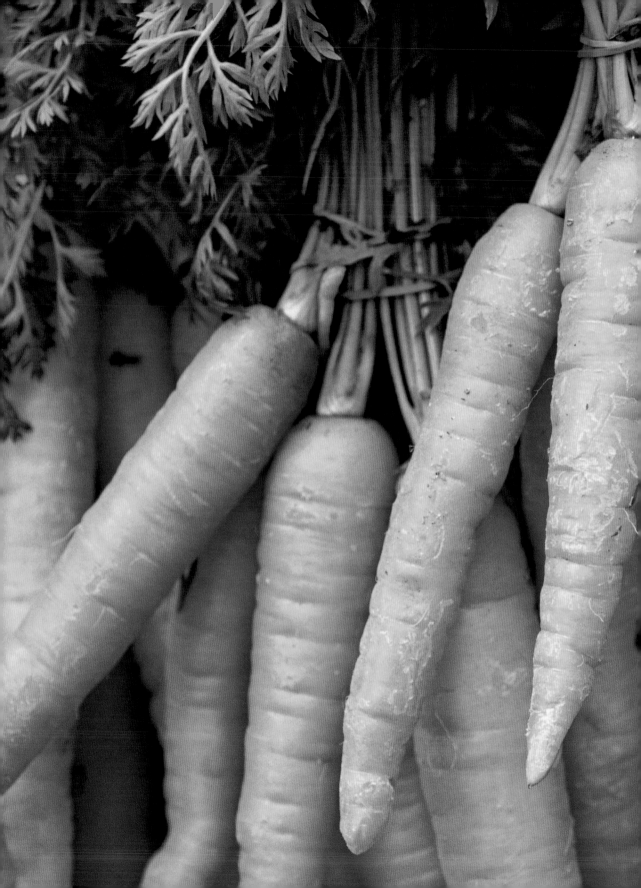

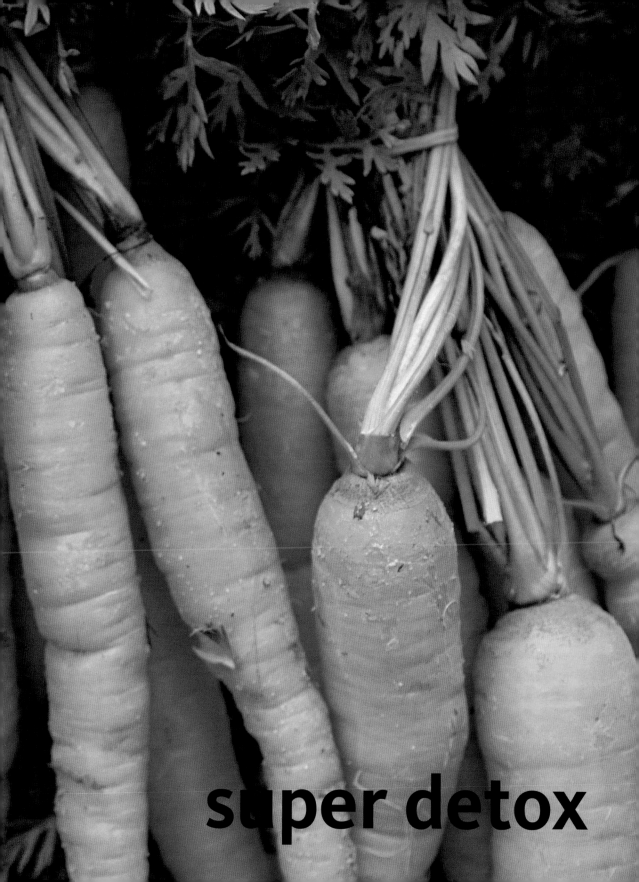

super detox

energy detox

This is a simple, energizing, 24-hour plan, but you will feel more comfortable and it will work more effectively if you start preparing 24 hours before you do the fast. During this time avoid all animal protein and stick to a pretty light diet of just fruit, salad, and vegetables. Make sure that you consume at least 6 cups of plain water and start cutting down on your coffee consumption to reduce the probability of a miserable headache by the time you finish the 24-hour fast. At bedtime the day before, use one of the natural bulk laxatives such as flaxseed or psyllium seeds.

As with any serious fast, even if it is for only 24 hours, it's best to do it when you can have the day at home so that you get plenty of rest. As long as they're in reasonable health, you'll probably cope with it at work, but most of my patients have found that it's not as easy as they think—especially when it comes to getting irritable with your colleagues, shouting down the telephone, and making poor decisions by the end of the day.

It's important that you consult your own family doctor before starting even the simplest 24-hour detox if you have any underlying medical problems that could contraindicate fasting, or if you are taking prescribed medication that should not be used on an empty stomach.

on waking: A large glass of hot water with a thick slice of organic unwaxed lemon.

breakfast: Another glass of hot water with lemon and the juice of 1 small pineapple (peeled).

mid-morning drink: Another glass of hot water with lemon.

midday: Juice of 4 carrots, 1 small sweet potato, and 2 beets – preferably with their leaves – followed by a mug of ginseng tea.

mid-afternoon drink: Another glass of hot water with lemon.

early evening: Juice of 1 mango (stoned), 2 kiwi fruit, 1 pawpaw, 1 peach (stoned), followed by a large mug of raspberry-leaf tea.

late evening: Juice of 4 carrots, 3 apples, and 2 celery sticks (with leaves).

bedtime drink: Large mug of chamomile tea sweetened with a teaspoon of organic honey.

throughout the day: You should drink at least another 4 cups of liquid; this can be more hot water and lemon, plain water, or any herbal tea but without milk, sugar, or honey. Avoid normal tea, coffee, and even decaffeinated coffee, as there will still be residual caffeine and several hundred other chemicals that you are better off without during this detox.

Diet notes

You can expect to develop a headache by midday and it will come on even earlier if you are a serious coffee drinker. More than 4 to 6 cups of coffee daily means that you will be pretty addicted to the caffeine, and headache is the first symptom of caffeine withdrawal.

During the next 24 hours you'll feel much more comfortable if you stick to a fairly light diet: vegetables, fruit, fish, and eggs would be best. Certainly you should avoid meat, poultry, game, and all processed foods manufactured from these three. Keep dairy products to a minimum; a little plain yogurt is okay, but keep away from cream and cheese.

The next morning, eat a banana and a large bunch of grapes for your breakfast and give your system a boost with a mug of lemon and ginger tea sweetened with 1 teaspoon of organic honey. Then, as normal, stick to a meat-free and refined-carbohydrate-free plan for the next 36 hours or so.

Thanks to the high natural sugar content of the juices, you won't feel as lethargic as you might with some of the other detox plans, in this section, but it's still best to do this on your day off so you can put your feet up.

radiance detox

If you want to look radiant on the outside, you need to be radiant on the inside, too. But there's no doubt that a combination of both gives you super radiance, with glowing skin, shining hair, and perfect nails. If you've looked in the mirror and think your radiance is on the wane, then you probably need a 24-hour radiance detox. Hopefully this will give you a chance to improve your long-term eating habits, too.

If cooking in your household means ready-meals from the supermarket, pot noodles, Chinese takeouts and instant soup, then it's not surprising that your skin is less than radiant. It's important to understand that skin is the biggest organ of the body and it's responsible for the elimination of many waste products.

It really doesn't matter if you do this 24-hour radiance detox because you've just had a weekend of total overindulgence or as part of your regular radiance routine. Whatever the reason, it's worth the effort – as you will soon see for yourself.

This detox is a short, sharp shock to the system and you'll find it much easier if you are at home and able to rest and take things gently. As long as you're reasonably fit, you will be able to manage it while you're at work – but you certainly won't enjoy it as much. Personally I've always found that my patients derive maximum benefit from this fast when they don't do it on a working day.

It's important that you consult your family doctor before starting even the simplest 24-hour detox if you have an underlying medical problem that means you shouldn't fast, or if you are taking prescribed medication that should not be used on an empty stomach.

on waking: A large glass of hot water with a slice of organic unwaxed lemon.

breakfast: Another glass of hot water with lemon. Juice together 2 large carrots, 2 large sweet apples, 1 inch (3/4 in) fresh gingerroot, then mix with the juice of 2 freshly squeezed oranges. A mug of lime-blossom tea.

mid-morning drink: Another glass of hot water with lemon.

midday: Juice 8 large ripe tomatoes, 2 scallions (with green parts), 10 basil leaves, and 1 garlic clove followed by a cup of nettle tea.

mid-afternoon drink: Another glass of hot water with lemon.

early evening: Juice of 1 large mango (stoned), 4 kiwi fruit, 1 medium pineapple (peeled), followed by a large mug of nettle tea.

late evening: Juice of 4 large carrots, 4 medium beets (preferably with leaves), 6 sage leaves rolled together.

bedtime drink: Large mug of lime-blossom tea sweetened with a teaspoon of organic honey.

throughout the day: You should drink at least another 4 cups of liquid; this can be more hot water and lemon, plain water, or any herbal tea but without milk, sugar, or honey. Avoid normal tea, coffee, and even decaffeinated coffee, as there will still be residual caffeine and several hundred other chemicals that you are better off without during this detox.

Diet notes

You can expect to develop a headache by midday and it will come on even earlier if you are a serious coffee drinker. More than 4 to 6 cups of coffee daily means that you will be pretty addicted to the caffeine, and headache is the first symptom of caffeine withdrawal.

During the next 24 hours you'll feel much more comfortable if you stick to a fairly light diet: vegetables, fruit, fish, and eggs would be best. Certainly you should avoid meat, poultry, game, and all processed foods manufactured from these three. Keep dairy products to a minimum; a little plain yogurt is okay, but keep away from cream and cheese.

The next morning, eat a banana and a large bunch of grapes for your breakfast and give your system a boost with a mug of lemon and ginger tea sweetened with 1 teaspoon of organic honey. Then, as normal, stick to a meat-free and refined-carbohydrate-free plan for the next 36 hours or so.

brain-boost detox

Living in the 24-hour, seven days a week society is not only a drain on physical resources, but it also rapidly exhausts your mental reserves too. The constant situation of heightened awareness and overproduction of adrenaline leads to a sure reduction in reserves of sugar, iron, and B vitamins. Add this to our heavy dependence on convenience foods, takeouts and artificial stimulants such as caffeine, nicotine, and alcohol, and the optimum performance of the brain is in serious jeopardy. Another major factor in declining brain performance is the absence of sufficient omega-3 fatty acids in the modern diet, especially those derived from oily fish.

This 24-hour brain-boost detox is not a panacea, yet it will enable you to experience a probably long-forgotten clarity of thought, peace of mind, and sense of mental wellbeing.

It's important that you consult your family doctor before starting even the simplest 24-hour detox if you have any underlying medical problems that could contraindicate fasting or if you are taking prescribed medication that should not be used on an empty stomach.

on waking: A large glass of hot water with a slice of organic unwaxed lemon.

breakfast: Another glass of hot water with lemon, followed by a smoothie made from 3 juiced apples put into a blender with 2 bananas, 2 tablespoons of smooth peanut butter, and 2 cups soy milk.

mid-morning drink: Another glass of hot water with lemon.

midday: Juice of half a large pineapple (peeled), 2 ripe pears, 3 Cox's apples, a small bunch of seedless black grapes, and 2 teaspoons flaxseed oil, followed by a cup of ginseng tea.

mid-afternoon drink: Another glass of hot water with lemon.

early evening: A smoothie made from the juice of 3 kiwi fruit, 1 pomegranate, and 4 passion fruit, blended with $2/3$ cup skim milk, 4 oz mascarpone cheese, 2 teaspoons of ground flaxseeds, and 2 teaspoons of brewer's yeast powder. Follow this with a mug of sage tea: put 6 chopped sage leaves in a mug of boiling water, cover, leave for 10 minutes, then strain off the leaves.

late evening: 2 cups American Concord red grape juice: put in a saucepan with the peel from 1 lime, 1 cinnamon stick, 2 cloves, and 1 sprig of rosemary; warm through but don't boil. Sprinkle with ground walnuts.

bedtime drink: Large mug of chamomile tea sweetened with a teaspoon of organic honey.

throughout the day: You should drink at least another 4 cups of liquid and this can be more hot water and lemon, plain wate,r or any herbal tea but without milk, sugar, or honey. Avoid normal tea, coffee, and even decaffeinated coffee as there will still be residual caffeine and several hundred other chemicals that you are better off without during this detox.

Diet notes

You can expect to develop a headache by midday and it will come on even earlier if you are a serious coffee drinker. More than 4 to 6 cups of coffee daily means that you will be pretty addicted to the caffeine and headache is the first symptom of caffeine withdrawal.

The drinks used during this brain-boost detox are rich in essential fatty acids from the nuts, seeds, and flaxseed oil, as well as providing brain-boosting B vitamins and other essential oils from the herbs and spices.

During the next 24 hours you'll feel much more comfortable if you stick to a fairly light diet: vegetables, fruit, fish, and eggs would be best. Certainly you should avoid meat, poultry, game, and all processed foods manufactured from these three. Keep dairy products to a minimum; a little plain yogurt is okay, but keep away from cream and cheese.

total cleanse detox

This 24-hour cleansing detox fast is great if you've been overdoing booze, buns, and burgers, and is a useful seasonal cleanse for the beginning of spring, summer, fall and winter, just to set you up for the coming months.

No matter how much effort you put into healthy living, there are unavoidable and toxic pollutants all around us. They're in the air we breathe, on the food we eat; they're in household chemicals, detergents, cleaners, polishes, adhesives, paints, and varnishes. They're even in the fire retardants used in fabrics, soft furnishing, and carpets, as well as highly toxic residues in the garden, most of which come from the arsenic used as a wood preservative. When it rains, arsenic salts leach from the lumber into the soil, they get on your shoes and you tread them through the house.

This simple regime is easy to fit into your daily schedule, though it's best to try it on a non-working day. If you're in reasonably good health, there's no reason why you can't do it on a work day, but the greatest benefit will come if you can get plenty of rest during this 24 hours.

It's important, however, that you consult your family doctor before starting even the simplest 24-hour detox if you have any underlying medical problems that could contraindicate fasting, or if you are taking prescribed medication that should not be used on an empty stomach.

on waking: A large glass of hot water with a slice of organic unwaxed lemon.

breakfast: Another glass of hot water with lemon and the juice of 1 orange, 1 grapefruit, and 1 lemon diluted 50/50 with hot water.

mid-morning drink: Another glass of hot water with lemon.

midday: Juice of 6 tomatoes and 4 sticks of celery (with their leaves) followed by a cup of green tea.

mid-afternoon drink: Another glass of hot water with lemon.

early evening: Juice of half a pineapple and 4 kiwi fruit, followed by a large mug of ginger tea: grate 2.5cm (1 in) peeled fresh gingerroot into a mug, add boiling water, cover, and leave for 10 minutes, strain, add 1 teaspoon of organic honey and sip slowly.

late evening: Juice 4 oranges and stir in 2 teaspoons of ground walnuts.

bedtime drink: A large mug of chamomile tea sweetened with a teaspoon of organic honey.

throughout the day: You should drink at least another liter (36 fl oz) of liquid and this can be more hot water and lemon, plain water, or any herbal tea, but without milk, sugar or honey. Avoid regular Indian tea, coffee and even decaffeinated coffee, as there will still be residual caffeine and several hundred other chemicals that you are better off without during this detox.

Diet notes

You can expect to develop a headache by midday and it will come on even earlier if you are a serious coffee drinker. More than 4 to 6 cups of coffee daily means that you will be pretty addicted to the caffeine and headache is the first symptom of caffeine withdrawal.

During the next 24 hours you'll feel much more comfortable if you stick to a fairly light diet: vegetables, fruit, fish and eggs would be best. Certainly you should avoid meat, poultry, game and all processed foods manufactured from these three. Keep dairy products to a minimum; a little plain yogurt is okay, but keep away from cream and cheese.

The next morning, eat a banana and a large bunch of grapes for your breakfast and give your system a boost with a mug of lemon and ginger tea sweetened with 1 teaspoon of organic honey. Then, as normal, stick to a meat-free and refined-carbohydrate-free plan for the next 36 hours or so.

immunity diet

All the evidence shows that organically grown, freshly picked produce is substantially richer in essential nutrients than the commercially produced equivalents. Experts working in the field of clinical ecology believe that even the healthiest diet chosen from non-organic sources may be deficient in the micronutrients essential for the proper functioning of the immune system. For example, samples of oranges bought direct from an organic grower in California contained up to 180 mg of vitamin C, whereas those found in a supermarket that looked identical contained *not one single milligram* of this vitamin (a vital part of the body's defense mechanism).

Recent statistics show that 40 per cent of women between the ages of 18 and 34 had worryingly low intakes of iron, and that 90 per cent of 16- to 18-year-olds were not getting enough of this essential mineral in their diets. Even without obvious signs of anemia, a low intake of iron affects the oxygen-carrying capacity of the blood, on which every living cell depends if it's to maintain its protective immunity. Two other minerals commonly deficient in the Western diet are zinc and selenium, both of which play key roles in the overall human defense mechanism.

Everyone needs an adequate intake of the highly protective foods that boost immunity and help prevent disease—and we need them all the time. This need is even more important when you are going through periods of exceptional stress, an unusual increase in physical activities, during pregnancy, epidemics of colds and flu, or even after periods of serious overindulgence like exotic vacations and Christmas. All good, fresh, and especially organic produce builds immunity, but some foods are more valuable than others. The following should form a substantial part of your daily diet: fruits such as blueberries, raspberries, apricots, prunes, kiwi fruits and all the tropical varieties; vegetables such as cabbage and all its relatives, endive, leeks, onions, garlic, mushrooms, pumpkin, sweet potatoes and all the other root vegetables. Good grains are essential too, especially whole wheat, oats, brown rice and barley; you should also be eating almonds, walnuts, Brazil nuts, hazelnuts, and pumpkin, sesame and sunflower seeds; all beans, especially soy, and don't forget the lentils. Also add plain yogurt, goat and sheep milk and their cheeses, oily fish, organic meat and poultry, organic eggs, and all forms of game. Finally, rosemary, thyme, cinnamon and gingerroot are important herbs and spices.

breakfast:
As with the healing diet on page 136, breakfast is desperately important as it sets the tone for the rest of the day. Free-range eggs, baked beans on wholewheat toast, or even a broiled kipper (if you can face fish in the morning) would all make a perfect start. If you're a cereal-eater, porridge or granola with added dried fruits and ground flaxseeds is also fine.

breakfast drink:
Go for berry juice. Juice a selection of blueberries, blackberries, raspberries, strawberries, cranberries, loganberries—enough for a large glassful. This will provide you with protective and immune-boosting chemicals for the whole day.

mid-morning snack:
Wholewheat toast with a banana, peanut butter, and a drizzle of honey will do far more for your immune system than a doughnut or a Danish pastry.

mid-morning drink:
Mixed vegetable juice—not out of a can (which is full of salt), but make it yourself. If you have to take it to work, put it in a thermos with some ice to keep it cold and refreshing. Use any 4 veggies from carrot, celery, asparagus, beet, radishes, sweet potato, turnip, and spinach.

lunch:
If this is a light meal, try a mushroom and tomato omelet sprinkled with parsley and thyme; broiled sardines with a mixed salad, including a selection of nuts and seeds; or organic chicken livers sautéed with onion and garlic, and served with brown rice and a purée of carrot, squash and sweet potato.

lunchtime drink:
Juice of asparagus, broccoli, celery, carrot put in a blender with the flesh of a ripe avocado and $2/3$ cup goat milk.

mid-afternoon snack:
Tinned salmon, sardines, or tuna for the healing essential fatty acids; an organic chicken sandwich and a mixture of dried fruits and nuts, particularly Brazil nuts and walnuts; a portion of natural organic yogurt with a spoon of organic honey, sprinkled with ground flaxseeds, chopped walnuts, or pine nuts.

mid-afternoon drink:
Fresh juice made with 1 pawpaw, $1/2$ cup black currants, $1/2$ cup red currants, $2/3$ cup blackberries, a handful of black grapes, and the flesh of 1 small butternut squash.

evening meal:
Homemade chicken soup; squash soup or spring vegetable soup (depending on season); any sort of organic meat: steak, cutlets, roast, or a slow-cooked bean and root vegetable casserole with at least 2 green vegetables; fresh fruit and some goat or sheep cheese.

evening drink:
Digestive juice made with 2 garlic cloves, 1 inch peeled gingerroot, 8 fresh mint leaves, 1 small leek, a few dark-green cabbage leaves, and 4 carrots. Serve sprinkled with ground caraway seeds.

bedtime drink:
A mug of *Melissa* (lemon-balm) tea with a teaspoon of organic honey.

healing diet

Most cookery books written before the 1960s included a whole section of recipes for invalids and the sickroom. Sadly, convalescence seems to be a luxury of the past, and healing is often pushed aside in the interests of economy, convenience, and prescription drugs. But what false economy this is – in the long term, it results in relapse, infection, and even more serious illness.

Convalescence was a time for healing and meant a few quiet days by the winter fire, summer afternoons in a garden deck chair or sitting on the seafront; with regular tonics, breakfast in bed, healing soups, and nourishing treats from the kitchen. The rush and bustle of modern life has dispatched convalescence to distant memory, and the priority these days is to get out of the sickbed, away from the hospital, and back to work as quickly as possible.

Modern medicine has become the search for the magic bullet, a remedy for every symptom and a treatment for every disease, all with total disregard of the holistic needs of the patient. You may think that a few extra days at home after a bout of flu is a waste of time, but in fact it wastes far less time than going back too soon, infecting all your colleagues and ending up back in bed with an even worse attack of flu and the risk of your already diminished immune system falling foul of an even worse infection such as pneumonia or TB.

The appropriate diet that will make sure that your body gets enough of the essential nutrients for the healing process is absolutely vital if you want to be restored to optimum and long-lasting good health. In this simple outline of a healing diet, you'll find lists of specific foods with the greatest healing properties, as well as recipes for super juices, drinks, and smoothies that will aid the healing process and help you back to better health as soon as possible. This is the time to regenerate and renew your body's healing powers; to replace, restore and repair the resulting damage and, as you've seen in the previous section, to rebuild your natural immunity.

In this healing situation, you need to avoid very large, heavy, and high-fat meals, that your body will find difficult to deal with. The secret is to eat four modest meals a day, interspersed with healing snacks and drinks.

breakfast:
This is almost the most important meal you'll eat as it is literally "breaking your fast." It should always include one of the healing super-grains such as oats, barley, or millet, so begin with granola, porridge, or millet flakes with the addition of some fresh berries, slivered almonds, and ground flaxseeds. Combine all this with natural plain yogurt. Alternatively, have some free-range eggs, wholewheat toast, and a small bunch of grapes. Your healing breakfast drink should be a juice made from a handful of white seedless grapes, 2 pears, 1 apple and 2 kiwi fruit, mixed with 2 freshly squeezed oranges.

mid-morning snack:
A few prunes and dried apricots with fresh walnuts, almonds, and pine kernels.

mid-morning drink:
A smoothie made from a small carton of plain yogurt, the flesh of 1 large mango, and 6 tablespoons of buttermilk.

lunch:
Any sort of oily fish, free-range chicken, or goat cheese, with a salad of raw beet, celery, carrot, baby spinach leaves with a walnut oil and lemon juice dressing sprinkled with sesame seeds.

lunchtime drink:
Juice together a large bunch of white seedless grapes, a handful of watercress, 1/2 cucumber and 6 dark-red plums, pits removed.

mid-afternoon snack:
A slice of simple homemade teabread made with calming chamomile tea, chopped dried dates for blood-building iron, and extra protein from the egg.

mid-afternoon drink:
A super healing juice made by juicing 3 large carrots, 2 apples, and 2 beets. This is a real blood-building tonic with healing betacarotenes from the carrots, natural sugars and protective chemicals in the apple, and an energy boost from the natural sugar in all 3 ingredients.

early evening snack:
Scrambled eggs with smoked salmon; lightly curried soup made from parsnip, rutabaga, and turnip; fresh asparagus with a little melted butter; a Belgian endive spear, halved, spread with goat cheese, sprinkled with oregano, drizzled with olive oil, and baked for 15 minutes.

early evening drink:
Healing lemonade: juice 1 large carrot, 12 radishes, 2 apples, and 1 small beet, then add the juice and zest of 1 lemon and combine with sparkling mineral water. This is a healing and liver-cleansing combination that is rich in vitamins A and C and natural energy.

drink yourself better

condition	superjuice	effect	dose
Acne	Cress to Impress, p 21	Provides carotenoids that are great for skin	4 glasses a week
AMD	The Gardener's Tonic, p 33	Highly protective carotenoids	2 glasses a week
Anemia	Love in a Glass, p 91	Rich in iron and zinc	1 glass daily for 2 weeks, then 1 a week
Anxiety	Bounce Back, p 57	Soothing basil and calming celery for nerves	As required
Arthritis	Welsh Wizard, p 16	Anti-inflammatory, pain-relieving, and energizing	At least 4 glasses a week
Asthma	Purple Lady, p 37	Nourishes lung tissue, protects against infection	1 glass daily
Back pain	Joint Pack, p 20	Anti-inflammatory, diuretic, pain-relieving	1 glass daily
Bronchitis	Celery Surprise, p 43	Antibacterial and decongesting	2 glasses daily during infectio
Catarrh	New Spring Clean Tonic, p 44	Decongestant, mucous membrane protector	1 glass daily when needed, 2 glasses a week as preventati
Chilblains	Hot Tom, p 81	Stimulates circulation, dilates peripheral blood vessels	2–3 glasses a week during winter
Cholesterol	Fast Tox, p 45	Stimulates bowel function and reduces cholesterol	At least 3 glasses a week
Chronic fatigue	Liquid Muscle, p 116	Instant and slow-release energy boosts vitality	1 glass daily
Circulation problems	Potato Protector, p 80	Stimulates circulation and helps to protect the heart	1 glass on alternate days
Colds	Beat the Bugs, p 117	Provides a huge dose of vitamin C, protective antioxidants, and anti-bacterial agents	2 glasses a day throughout cold, and for 2 days afterwards
Constipation	Tooty Fruity, p 38	Gently laxative	1 glass at bedtime
Cough	Celery Surprise, p 43	Antibacterial and decongesting	1 glass daily until better
Cramp	Sweet William, p 13	Potassium from banana is cramp-preventative	1 glass in the evening for nigh cramp, or before sports

condition	superjuice	effect	dose
Cystitis	Cranberry Source, p 76	Antibacterial, specifically protects against bugs that cause cystitis	1 glass daily during infection; 3 glasses a week for prevention
Depression	Perfect Balance, p 49 Ancient Wisdom, p 50	Provides lots of B vitamins and mood-enhancing phytoestrogens	1 glass of either, daily
Dermatitis	Tutti Frutti, p 38	Provides betacarotene for healthy skin and vitamin C to help prevent skin infections	3 glasses a week
Diarrhea	Fast Tox, p 45	Provides prebiotic food for friendly bugs and is a gentle liver cleanser	1 or 2 glasses daily as required
Eczema	Mangavo, p 86	Provides skin-healing vitamins A and E	1 glass daily until clear
Fever	Klever Kiwis, p 51	Provides Protective anti-oxidants, healing enzymes and vitamin C	2 glasses a day until temperature falls
Fibrositis	Pis en Lit, p 111	Strongly diuretic. Eliminates pain-causing uric acid	2–3 glasses a week
Flatulence	Celery Surprise, p 43	Provides anti-flatulence essential oils from fennel	Half a glass after meals
Fluid retention	Pis en Lit, p 111	Strongly diuretic to eliminate fluid	1 glass daily, when necessary
Fractures	Liquid Muscle, p 116	Provides lots of calcium and other minerals to speed bone healing	1 glass daily
Gallstones	Fast Tox, p 45	Radishes specifically stimulate gall bladder and liver function	1 glass daily
Gingivitis	Oracle Juice, p 68	Antiseptic, antifungal, and lots of gum healing nutrients	1 glass daily, as long as necessary
Gout	Joint Pack, p 20	Provides bioflavonoids, potassium, vitamin C, anti-inflammatory and specific uric acid-reducing properties	1 glass daily during attacks, 2 glasses a week for prevention
Halitosis	Celery Surprise, p 64	Antibacterial. Also provides healing enzymes, and breath-freshening essential oils	1 glass daily, as required
Hayfever	Tropical Treasure, p 25	Provides masses of vitamin C. For extra protection, add a tablespoon of locally produced honey	1 glass daily
Headache	Memories are Made of This, p 61	Provides essential fatty acids, vitamins C and E.	1 glass daily until headaches recede, then twice a week

condition	superjuice	effect	dose
Heart disease	Oracle Juice, p 68	Provides antioxidants to protect against heart diseases	1 glass daily
Heartburn	The Perfect Pair, p 30	Soothing pectin. Add a sprig of mint for antacid effect	1 glass as required
Hepatitis	Purple Lady, p 37	Strawberries are effective liver cleansers	2 glasses weekly
Herpes	Citrus Slimmer, p 108	Provides antiviral vitamin C and bioflavonoids	1 glass daily during attacks, 2 glasses weekly for protectio
Hypertension	Oracle Juice, p 68	Provides antioxidants to protect against heart and circulatory diseases	1 glass daily
Impotence	Mangavo, p 86	Rich in vitamin E and betacarotene for improved function	2 or 3 glasses a week
Indigestion	Citrus Symphony, p 26	Stimulates digestive juices to improve digestion	1 glass as required
Infections	Beat the Bugs, p 117	Rich in natural antibacterials and vitamins to boost the body's defences	1 glass daily during illness
Infertility	Mangavo, p 86 Love in a Glass, p 91	Vitamin E, betacarotene and helpful enzymes in Mangavo; zinc, iron and stimulants in Love in a Glass	alternate 1 glass of each daily
Influenza	Tropical Treasure, p 25	Provides soothing enzymes for aches and pains, masses of vitamin C, and betacarotene for resistance	1 or 2 glasses daily until you recover
Insomnia	Peaceful Pears, p 62	Provides natural sleep-inducing essential oils in lavender	1 glass before bed
Joint pain	Joint Pack, p 20	Anti-inflammatory, and rich in bioflavonoids and potassium	At least 4 glasses a week
Kidney problems	Waterfall 2, p 105	Diuretic and protective	1 glass daily
Laryngitis	Welsh Wizard, p 16	Antibacterial volatile oils from the garlic, and traditional voice benefits from leeks	1 glass daily
Motion and early morning sickness	Watermelon and Coconut Countdown, p 79	Volatile oils in ginger prevent sickness	1 glass before travelling or as required
Mouth ulcers	Celery Surprise, p 43	Rich in healing natural antibacterials and enzymes	1 glass as required. Take regularly for prevention
Obesity	The Three P's, p 106 Nutmeg Nectar, p 110	Sustaining to keep you going between meals	1 glass as a replacement for o meal daily

condition	superjuice	effect	dose
Osteoporosis	Boney M, p 123	Contains calcium and other beneficial natural plant hormones	1 glass daily
PMS	The Moody Swinger, p 54	Essential oils are calming and mood-enhancing. Also diuretic so reduces bloating	1 glass each day before and during the first 2 days of period
Prostate problems	Hot Tom, p 81	Protective lycopene that acts as a prostate protector	1 glass daily until symptoms improve, then 3 times a week
Psoriasis	Mangavo, p 86	Provides skin-healing vitamins A and E	1 glass daily
Raynaud's syndrome	Watermelon and Coconut Countdown, p 79	Betacarotene improves the quality of blood vessels, while the ginger stimulates circulation	1 glass daily during cold weather
Restless legs	Blue Strawberries, p 32	Contains iron, anti-oxidants, and natural anti-inflammatories	1 glass before bed as required
Rheumatism	Joint Pack, p 20	Anti-inflammatory, diuretic and pain-relieving	At least 4 glasses a week
Seasonal Affective Disorder (SAD)	Hot Mango, p 40	Provides B vitamins, vitamin A, potassium and iron to help this condition	1 glass daily during the winter
Shingles	Welsh Wizard, p 16	Antivirals in the leek and garlic	1 glass when required
Sinusitis	Hot Mango p 40 New Spring Clean Tonic p 44	Stimulates cleansing in the sinuses	Daily when needed, 2 glasses a week as preventative
Stomach ulcers	Tropical Sport, p 120	Healing enzymes from the pineapple and mango, and antacids in the bananas and coconut milk. Use manuka rather than Greek honey	1 glass daily
Thyroid problems	Stir-fry Cocktail, p 101	Provides iodine, vitamin A, and other preventative nutrients	2 glasses a week (the sake is optional)
Tonsillitis	Tropical Treasure, p 25	Full of protective antibacterial nutrients, and especially throat-soothing enzymes	3 or 4 small glasses daily

what does "orac" mean?

Medicine has conquered many infectious diseases. You can have a new heart or hip, and drugs can keep you mobile as your joints stiffen. However, much of this is papering over the cracks. Aging is a relentless march of nutritional deficiencies, and in spite of the many medical advances we have achieved, the relevance of nutrition and its anti-aging function is often overlooked.

You can slow down and even reverse many of the body's natural aging processes. You'll not only feel and look better, but you'll gain enormous protection against the scourges of heart disease and some cancers. All you have to do is eat more of the specific foods that are richest in nature's defensive chemicals: antioxidants.

At the core of the ageing process is a group of chemicals called "free radicals," produced mainly when the body burns up oxygen. We're also subject to free radicals that get into our system from outside, caused by smoking, environmental pollution, radiation, too much sunlight, and irritant chemicals that make contact with our skin. Free radicals destroy body cells. Our only protection are antioxidants, which attack and neutralize free radicals. If you eat right, your level of antioxidants will be more than a match for free radicals.

So where do you find the foods richest in these miracle chemicals? At the street market, your local store, the supermarket, or even in your own back yard. They are present in simple, everyday, inexpensive fruits and vegetables. Of course, all fruits and vegetables are good sources of vitamins like A, C, and E, but those that are deeply colored (dark green, deep red, purple, yellow, and bright orange) tend to have the highest levels of vitamins and minerals.

The US Department of Agriculture Human Nutrition Research Center on Aging at Tufts University has invented a method of testing the antioxidant strength of food by measuring its oxygen radical absorbance capacity (ORAC). The table on this page shows the fruits and vegetables with the highest ORAC scores. The numbers below represent the ORAC units in $1/2$ cup of food. Most experts agree that getting between 3,000 and 5,000 ORAC units a day has a huge impact on the body's ability to fight off free radicals, and reduce the risk of damage and aging.

High-ORAC fruits and vegetables	Units per $1/2$ cup
Prunes	5,570
Raisins	2,830
Blueberries	2,400
Blackberries	2,036
Garlic	1,939
Curly kale	1,770
Cranberries	1,750
Strawberries	1,540
Spinach	1,260
Raspberries	1,220
Brussels sprouts	980
Plums	949
Alfalfa sprouts	930
Broccoli	890
Beet	840
Avocado	782
Oranges	750
Black grapes	739
Red sweet pepper	710
Cherries	670
Kiwi fruit	602
Pink grapefruit	483
Onions	450
Corn	400
Eggplant	390

index

144 index